THE NATURAL LAWS
OF HEALTHFUL LIVING

The Bio-Nature Health Rhythm Program

Other books by the author:

Helping Your Health with Enzymes

Magic Minerals: Key to Better Health

*The Natural Way to Health Through
Controlled Fasting*

*Carlson Wade's Gourmet Health
Foods Cookbook*

Natural and Folk Remedies

THE NATURAL LAWS
OF HEALTHFUL LIVING

The Bio-Nature Health Rhythm Program

by CARLSON WADE

Foreword by
H. W. HOLDERBY, M.D.

PARKER PUBLISHING COMPANY, INC.
West Nyack, N.Y.

Printed in the United States of America
ISBN-0-13-610139-9
B & P

DEDICATION

To Nature—The Healing Lawgiver

FOREWORD BY A DOCTOR OF MEDICINE

This new and timely book by Carlson Wade, a brilliant scientific writer, details many of the methods of natural healing that are at our disposal. These are not expensive methods, but their truths are worth fortunes to us in longer and healthier and more productive lives.

PILLS, PILLS, PILLS. It seems we have become a nation of pill takers. About 28 times in every second a prescription is being filled by a white-coated pharmacist at one of the approximately sixty thousand drugstores in the United States. The staggering cost of these pink, purple, white, yellow, green, red, black, orange, gray and rainbow pills amounts to about $4 billion dollars annually.

Headache? Take a pill. Indigestion, insomnia, depressed or tense, take a pill. We seem to be looking for a color-coded new world. A green pill for anxiety, a yellow pill for sleep, an orange pill for frustration, a purple pill for indigestion, a white pill for a headache, a gray pill for a bad day at the office, a red one to direct this traffic and a black pill when all else fails.

We are standing at the drugstore counters of America, trying to buy good health. We are like animals standing before a water trough, thinking perhaps that the drugstore is the spot from whence all health blessings flow.

Millions of Americans take pills on their own on their doctors' advice, every day, for every ill from an upset stomach to an upset psyche. We consume tons of drugs a day in our headlong pursuit of health by the drug route. Would you believe we Americans average swallowing 23½ tons of aspirin daily?

We seem to share a childlike unquestioning faith that the answer to all our health problems lies in a pill, and that if we do not have a pill for every problem today, the drug companies will come with an answer tomorrow. When will we learn that drugs do not cure disease?

Now, however, many thoughtful leaders of the United States, medical profession are having second thoughts about America's and the world's pill-mania. We are seeing an epidemic of pill-caused diseases. We worry about the silent and deadly effects of long-term pill taking. Carl Linnaeus (1707-1788) said, "To live by medicine is to live horribly."

We have taken mountains of pills and lakes of liquid medicines trying to cure our diseases, when we should know that drugs act by interfering with the physiological functioning of the body. We are creating a nightmare world of drug-induced diseases.

People need to be taught that drugs do not cure disease. It is true that they sometimes afford present relief, and the patient appears to recover as the result of their use. This is because nature has sufficient vital force to expel the poison and correct the condition that caused the disease. Health is recovered in spite of the drug. But in most cases the drug only changes the form and location of the disease. Often the effect of the poison seems to be overcome for a time, but the results remain in the system, and work great harm at some later period. By the use of poisonous drugs, many bring upon themselves a life-long illness, and many lives are lost that might be *saved by natural methods of healing.*

The drug commercials are so loud, harsh and incessant, that they often jam the channels of communication. The bewildered physician prescribes by suggestion and not from information.

Too many physicians are getting writer's cramps making out prescriptions for patients who demand them, forgetting the story of the physician who handed a prescription to a patient saying, "Here, have this filled quickly, while it is still a remedy."

It is stated that when a young physician starts practice, he has 20 pills for each disease, but the doctor who has been at it for many years has one pill for 20 diseases.

I heartily recommend this new book to each of you. Natural methods of healing are the only roads that lead to good health; all others are detours.

H. W. Holderby, M.D.

WHAT THIS BOOK
CAN DO FOR YOU

As an editor, reporter and writer for many years on health, I have repeatedly been asked by physicians, practitioners of various other healing arts, and many readers, to compile a set of all-Natural laws that would help promote healing and rejuvenation of the body and mind. While doing research for my medical and health articles and books, and while interviewing leading health authorities in all branches of the healing arts, I began to gather a treasure of drugless healing methods that reportedly restored good health and reversed the "aging clock." As more and more of these drugless healing laws were given to me by consultation with health authorities, I began to compile a *system of natural laws* that were based on all-Natural healing methods and were easy to follow for rebuilding and regaining abundant good health. Many health authorities who saw my compilation urged me to prepare a book on these natural laws. They were enthusiastic about such a book because it would fill a modern health need and bridge a gap between man and Natural Laws for health.

This book is a unique guide for everyone who seeks to get more out of living and enjoy a greater measure of vigorous health and younger appearance. All this can be done without drugs or potentially harmful medication and chemicalized pills or their side effects.

The natural laws and how to use them have been arranged for your speedy reference. Easy to follow, in the privacy of your own home, the programs offer benefits for every member of the family.

How to build a more youthful skin, a "trouble-free" digestion, dynamic mental stamina, protection against allergies, supple and youthful arteries, healing sleep, and an herbal mini-encyclopedia are just a few samples comprising the range of health benefits for you in this book.

The many natural laws are listed in simple arrangement to help you easily plan your complete program to build good health. Some natural laws require ordinary fruits and vegetables in certain combination. Other natural laws call for just water. Still many more call for simple self- massage to help alert and revitalize sluggish circulation processes. The unique benefit here is that the natural laws are so *surprisingly simple,* requiring a few moments, with *no* unnecessary expense (many are totally free!), that the reader will be amazed at the "instant" programs By means of many reported case histories throughout the book you will discover the benefit of all-Nature healing that worked so well for other people who gladly discarded drugs and medications. Case history after case history attest to the beneficial operation of Nature's laws for helping you super-charge your body with youthful vitality.

Let these natural laws work for you to give you the daily vitality and youthful health that you deserve for yourself for more dynamically healthful living.

Carlson Wade

CONTENTS

1

HOW TO TAP THE NATURAL SOURCES OF REJUVENATED HEALTH WITHIN YOUR BODY

Your body is the most perfect, healthful and best put-together mechanism ever created. Within your body, Nature placed a million dollar "wellspring" of self-healing and self-rejuvenation. This bubbling source of revitalization serves to give a glow of youth to your skin, a smooth joint flexibility, a feeling of digestive satisfaction, and a mind that remains alert even when calendar years may suggest otherwise. All of these "always young, always healthy" treasures have been given to you by Nature right within your own body. The prime purpose of this book is to show you how you can tap these hidden "wellsprings" of bubbling health and emotion-energy by using the secrets of Nature.

Magic Self-Cleansing Food

Although she was in her very early 40's, Beth R. looked much older. She walked with a stooped gait, appeared vague and listless, was prone to frequent cold catching. Beth R. complained of feeling "stuffed up." She was embarrassed about her recurring constipation. If ever anyone suffered from "irregularity," it was Beth R. She took commercial laxatives, and the harsh cathartic salts and abrasive chemicals had so weakened her intestinal-digestive tract that she was addicted to them! Because of this inner clogging, her digestive system was malfunctioning. Precious nutrients to nourish the bloodstream, hormonal system, and arterial network were choked and unable to provide life-giving fuel. Small wonder that her entire health began to decline.

How a Return to Nature Created Abundantly Healthful Living. Beth R. thought she had tried everything until she read an advertisement that offered a drug-composed laxative with the promise that it had "some natural ingredients." This gave Beth an idea. Why not "try Nature" — but entirely, and not in combination with artificial patent medicines? She started reading about the healing power of ordinary foods and came across a simple and all-natural home "morning broth" that was rich in the precious nutrients needed to unlock her clogged insides. She would try it, she resolved.

MAGIC SELF–CLEANSING MORNING BROTH. The program was so simple, Beth wondered if it would work. Yet, Beth would soon learn (as will you!) that Nature is surprisingly simple in providing blessed relief and home folk healers. All Nature requires of you is one item — *cooperation.* Beth would cooperate with Nature by preparing this Magic Self-Cleansing Morning Broth:

Mix together ground whole-wheat, a small chopped onion, a crushed clove of garlic. Boil in water. When bubbly, add some chopped parsley and two tablespoons of olive oil. Let boil for a **few** moments. Remove. Pour into cup and sip slowly. You may have a slice of crisp whole grain bread with this Morning Broth, and it may be considered a nourishing breakfast.

This all-Nature broth is a rich source of vitalic-minerals that exert an electrolytic reaction within the intestinal canal to help unblock the clogging and restore natural regularity. It is most beneficial when taken first thing in the morning.

Beth R. had agreed to give up all of her commercial laxatives and to further eliminate all artificial bleached white baked foods and sugar-containing foods. This would give the Magic Self-Cleansing Morning Broth a complete free rein to exert its inner scrubbing.

Nature Washes the Insides and Creates an Outside Sparkle. It took up to eight days before Beth R. was "regular." Furthermore, she felt so exhilarated; she was overjoyed with a feeling of youth and vitality. She felt good and she looked good. Her posture was straight, her skin texture was firm and healthful, she no longer feared catching cold upon the slightest little chill in the air. By washing the inside, Nature restored the health of the outside. Beth R. now could honestly and healthfully say that she loved life!

How This Book Offers Bonus-Plus Benefits

The unusual feature of this book is that you can follow nearly all of these programs and health secrets right in your own home! Many of the ingredients will be found in any kitchen pantry; many programs call for *no* equipment or devices and are ABSOLUTELY FREE! The most thrilling benefit of this book is that nearly all of the Nature-healers are *drugless*. It is the purpose of Nature to give you proper foods, proper free-form and instant exercises, healthful air and water healers, all created to help stir up your sluggish self-healing wellsprings – right within your body and your mind! As we progress, we shall discover the health building benefit of the underlying theme of Nature–*"Let food be your medicine!"*

By using the foods and programs of Nature to help rejuvenate and revitalize your body and your mind, you benefit in these ways:

1. *Freedom from drug dependence.* The drug habit can often be a lifetime addiction. Drugs and patent medicines may relieve symptoms, yet frequently fail to provide the corrective healing which is the miracle benefit of Nature. Many who complain of headaches, insomnia, nervous tension, joint stiffness, poor blood, become victims of lifetime drug dependence. The condition still remains and even becomes worse, while drugs enslave the user into a lifetime habit.

2. *Nature is free from side effects.* When utilizing an all-Nature food or program, there are no side effects as from drugs. Aspirins, for example, are known to cause internal

bleeding and hemorrhages. Certain cough medicines contain narcotics. Many prescription-only drugs offer temporary relief for the condition, yet will induce drowsiness, nausea, increased heartbeat, sallow skin and hair loss. These anti-Nature chemicals cause internal upheaval and may soothe symptoms on the one side, but cause serious side effects on the other. Nature is kind and gentle and so is her treasury of corrective healers.

3. *Nature is free for the taking.* The use of water, air, self-massage, easy-to-follow exercises, sunshine and bathing are all free for the taking. This is quite a contrast to the lifetime use of non-curative drugs that can cost a fortune in money and .unfulfilled hopes. Most of the corrective healers in this book are absolutely free. This is as much good news to you as the hope for restoring a corrective healing rhythm within yourself to put you in the circle of radiant health.

4. *Nature is a delicious way to build health.* Healthful foods, soothing broths, juicy good food combinations that taste as good as they heal! Nature offers a farm-fresh way to enjoy your food and enjoy healing through released nutrients at the same -time.

5. *Nature offers you complete privacy.* Many of the corrective healing programs of this book may be followed in the, complete privacy of your home. There are some foods and herbs you will need to acquire at a local supermarket or herbal pharmacy, but you will not be inconvenienced by having to search for unusual items. You may follow these programs in your own home at your leisure.

6. *Nature helps your entire family.* The unique benefit of this book is that it has something for every member of the family. A husband who is "too tired" or under tension, will find programs to put a natural energizer into his body mechanism in a matter of moments. A wife who complains of "aging skin" will discover how ordinary steam can flush out dirt-clogs of the pores and how raw juices can put youth into the "body envelope" that is the skin. Youngsters, whether boys or girls, are undergoing glandular changes. A nervous youngster can be a terror to himself and to his family! This book has all-natural

programs for helping youngsters — and adults — put happiness into their glands! Since the hormonal system rules vitality, energy, nervous temperament, physical characteristics and allergic symptoms, this is the precious "Fountain of Youth" that Nature can help bubble over with joyful health. Special emphasis on the glands is made in this book.

Two-Minute "Neck Rolling" Exercise for Headache Freedom

Louis B. was an accountant for a leading Eastern manufacturer. He loved his work, was slated for promotions, yet started making mistakes. This could have been costly had not a superior caught them and brought them to his attention. Louis B. now admitted that he was troubled with a feeling of "tightness" in the back of his neck. This made his eyesight blurred. Furthermore, he was troubled with recurring headaches that aspirins did not relieve. His work suffered as much as his health.

A co-worker suggested that he give up aspirins and try a series of two-minute "neck rolling" exercises.

Benefit of Simple "Neck Rolling." These all-natural exercises help relieve pressure on the cranial nerves and tissues and also help improve clogged circulation, which frequently is the cause of headaches. These following exercises helped Louis B. by opening up the interstices between the vertebrae, permitting circulation of all the neck and ear fluids.

BASIC NECK ROLLING EXERCISE. This calls for twisting, circling the head in a rolling motion, bending the head down to each shoulder, bending the neck forward and downward. Louis would do this for two minutes while sitting at his desk! It helped to free the kinks in his neck muscles and tissues and provided improved circulation. He found it helped ease some of his headache and, because it eased his back-of-the-neck tension, his eyesight improved.

TENSION-MELTING EXERCISE. But Louis B. was under tension; he worked extra long in an effort to gain the coveted promotion. To cope with a feeling of headache-tension, he followed this simple program that is best done at home:

This exercise helps give a healthful neck stretch and a good contraction to your tight neck muscles. You can do this on a bed, bench or table. Begin by lying on your back; let your head hang downward fully at the end. Now raise your head to the fullest upward forward position.

Repeat by lowering your head downward to lowest position possible with a little additional attempt to lower it farther, and then repeat the upward contraction.

VARIATION OF TENSION-MELTING EXERCISE. After a few repetitions, lie face down and do the reverse of the preceding exercise; that is, with your head protruding beyond the bench, let your head hang downward as far as possible, even attempting to stretch it a little farther, and then draw your head backward upward as far as possible and repeat.

Louis B. Finds Freedom from Headaches through Nature-Motions. It was necessary for Louis to do the preceding exercises every night as a means of loosening up the tensions of the day. He did exclaim that he slept better because of this inner freedom. He was no longer "all tied up in gnarled knots," which leads to insomnia. It took several weeks before the fluids of his body could flow unhindered. With a healthful circulation and corrective exercises, his headaches passed, his eyesight was sharper and—he got the coveted promotion. Credit Nature with a reward of gratitude.

How to Test Your Bio-Nature Health Rhythm

To reap the greatest benefit from this book, you need to establish a Bio-Nature Health Rhythm. The following test will help alert you to the need for the corrective and all-natural healers described in this book. Before you take this easy test (just a few moments of time can add up to a lifetime of health), note an important discovery of Bio-Nature Health Rhythm:

Heal the Body as a Whole. The secret of establishing an inner rhythm is to use Nature to create corrective healing *of the* *entire body.* The precious built-in high efficiency and longevity-endurance can be liberated and set into motion *only* when you create harmony *as a whole,* and not just as an assembly of separating aching parts. It is true that some of the programs are aimed directly at one particular health problem; but the success of the healing is related in direct proportion to the healing of the entire body.

How Healing of Parts Was Contrary to Nature. Marcia R., age 44, was able to resist chronic cold-catching, ease her coughing, stop her sniffling, when she made it a delicious practice to eat raw fruits in abundance. The rich store of tissue-building Vitamin C and precious bioflavonoids strengthened the capillaries and created cold resistance. She also drank herbal teas which were free from caffeine and tannic acids. This should have helped Marcia's health problem of chronic cold catching, but it was a healing of parts and soon failed.

What was wrong? Marcia loved sugary sweets and heavy desserts laced with syrups and confections. The high intake of devitalized and bleached sugar oxidized her precious supply of bioflavonoids and her resistance was lowered. She soon contracted a severe case of bronchitis that required prolonged and very costly hospitalization. It is hoped that Marcia R. will learn that healing is more successful if the *entire body* is renewed through all-Nature, as this book will describe.

HOW TO TAKE THIS SIMPLE TEST. Sit down at a comfortable table. On a piece of paper, score 10 for each *Yes.* Score 5 for each *Sometimes.* Score 1 for each *No.* At the end of this simple test, you will read how to score your health capacity.

Your Bio-Nature Health Rhythm Test

1. Are there times when you feel "heavy" or as though you have a "lump in the pit of the stomach" after a meal?
2. Do you have signs of aging on your skin? On the backs of your hands? Is your skin coloring less than satisfactory?
3. Are there some foods that you once could eat, but no longer eat because of digestive upset?
4. Do you find yourself fumbling for the correct words when

called upon to speak? Do you have occasional memory lapses? Are your thoughts rusty in comparison to what they were in times past?

5. Are you troubled with burning stomach, acid indigestion, hyperacidity that causes knife-like pains after a meal?

6. Are you embarrassed by constipation?

7. Are you troubled with seemingly uncontrollable personality changes? That is, are you temperamental? Do you get angry at the slightest provocation? Do simple things make you edgy? Do you get nervous if you have to wait in line? Are there times when you feel like yelling at someone for no apparent purpose?

8. Is tension getting the best of you? Are you becoming addicted to tranquilizers, headache remedies, assorted pills and capsules that give you a false sense of relaxation?

9. Troubled by recurring insomnia? Does it mean you are more tired when you awaken than when you go to sleep—if you can sleep?

10. Are you bothered with early morning back stiffness that has an arthritic stab of pain when you try to turn over in bed?

11. Are your fingers, elbows, joints, legs and toes, slowly becoming stiff and less flexible?

12. Bothered with rectal-bladder distress that calls for excessive bathroom trips?

13. Do you "lose your wind" when having to climb up more than a dozen steps?

14. Annoyed by cold hands and cold feet—even if the weather is comfortable or when you're indoors in a nice warm room?

15. Speaking about the weather—are you affected by climatic changes? Does a change trigger off bronchial disorders, nervous upset, feelings of depression?

16. Are there times when you just do not feel like eating? That is, do you have poor appetite?

17. Are you embarrassed by unsteadiness or clumsiness that may cause things to drop from your fingers even though you are certain you have a tight grip?

18. Do you have creeping sensations of "fog-bound moments" or a sensation of being alternately hot and cold, as in a

fever? This need not be a daily distress; rather, if it is a recurring problem, it should be noted as such.

19. Is it easy for you to get up from your chair or your bed or out of your bathtub?

20. (Be honest with this last question!) Are you overweight?

HOW TO SCORE:

"Yes" Answers. Between 0-100—Nature has created warning symptoms that the rhythm of your health is on a slow decline. *Between 100-150*—Nature is struggling to keep the vitals of your basic health but corrective healing is needed with no delays. *Between 150-200*—Nature is threatened with a losing battle since the Bio-Nature Health Rhythm is precariously tipped in the opposite direction.

"Sometimes" Answers. Between 0-30—Slight health decline that may continue downward if corrective methods are not utilized. *Between 30-50*—You are not getting the joy of life and health that Nature has waiting for you. The outlined programs of this all-Natural book should be applied with little further delay. *Between 50-100*—Health is slipping through your fingers, little by little. It may be reversed in time with utilization of natural health methods.

"No" Answers. Between 0-7—Occasional health problems should serve as signals to alert you to corrective healings. *Between 7-14*—You have a steady increase in upset Health Rhythm. To delay is to further upset the delicate natural balance. *Between 14-20*—You are pushing your luck too far. You may be on the brink of an increasing and insidiously slow health corrosion.

How This Book Will Help Promote Your Health Harmony

The methods, programs, natural food healers, herbal secrets, are all created for the purpose of helping to promote your overall health harmony. Bio-Nature will help you develop internal and external balance. The benefit is that Bio-Nature techniques as outlined in this book will create overall health harmony. The methods described release the hidden wellsprings of rejuvenation that have been placed within the body by Nature.

When you give your body the natural raw materials with which to regain, rebuild and replenish life and health, you then establish a rapport and communication with Bio-Nature Health Rhythm. It is to that goal that this book is dedicated.

Summary of Benefits:

1. Corrective healing is created by tapping the hidden million dollar "wellspring" of rejuvenation right within your own body.

2. The key to healthful living is in a cleansed digestive tract. The Magic Self-Cleansing Food helped Beth R. enjoy natural regularity without drugs. It gave her a new healthful lease on life.

3. Natural programs are drugless, free from addiction, free from side effects, often free for the taking, and a delicious way to build health.

4. Follow most of these health discoveries right in the privacy of your own home. There are benefits for every member of the family.

5. Simple "neck rolling" can end problems of chronic neck and head pain where aspirins only masked the symptoms and increased internal tensions.

6. Test your own health harmony and see how urgent it is for you to follow the ways of Nature.

7. The *entire body* must be Nature-tuned for overall healthy happiness. Treating parts may offer temporary relief but why settle for being half alive when you can be all alive! Create an alliance with Nature to stimulate healthful living, according to the easy-to-follow outlined programs of this book.

2

HOW TO USE RAW FOODS TO HELP NATURE REBUILD BODY AND MIND

Richard P. felt that each day was getting longer and longer. As a salesman, he was required to keep moving around and also to remain alert for customer questions and complaints. But Richard's nerves became brittle and his answers were sharp and offending. There were days when he could hardly remain on his feet for more than a short while. Once, when he felt the room spin and his heart pound in his throat, he decided that something was wrong.

Rather belatedly, he was completely examined. Healthwise, he should have been satisfactory. But dietwise, he was actually eating himself into premature aging. When asked about his eating, Richard said that most of his foods were cooked. He rarely ate anything raw; even juicy good fruit was eaten in a cooked form. This was the clue to his erratic behavior. He was put on a tasty but corrective eating program that called for an abundance of raw fruits and vegetables. It took several weeks for improvement to be seen, and then Richard P. felt young again. Life was well worth living.

Raw Foods—Nature's Staff of Life

The most valuable and precious natural law of abundantly healthful living is that raw foods are brimming with nutrients that can supercharge the body with rejuvenation. Fruits, vegetables, some grains, should be eaten *raw* to give the body the much-needed nutrients with which to build and rebuild the body and mind.

Raw Foods Are More Nutritious Than Cooked Foods

Raw foods are rich in the precious vitamins, minerals, enzymes, carbohydrates, natural fats that help create a healthful body and mind. Cooking causes depletion of the valuable fluids of the plant or grain; with them go also the natural flavors and aromas of the food. Digestibility is also lowered in cooked foods.

RAW FOODS NOURISH THE EYES AND SKIN. Uncooked fruits and vegetables are prime sources of Vitamins A and C, the two nutrients that serve to nourish the eyesight and the skin. Cooking processes dissolve these natural vitamins. Fresh raw fruits and vegetables are rich in these sight-and-skin-building nutrients.

RAW FOODS HELP ENRICH THE BLOODSTREAM. Precious minerals such as iron, copper calcium and phosphorous help feed the hemoglobin of the bloodstream and nourish the platelets of the red blood cells. These nutrients are abundant in uncooked fruits and vegetables. Cooking causes the minerals to be dissolved out and lost in cooking water that is discarded. To provide your bloodstream with the mineral nourishment required, eat fresh raw fruits and vegetables daily.

RAW FOODS ARE POWER SOURCES OF ENERGY. Ripe fruit should be eaten raw because it contains carbohydrates that consist almost entirely of easily digested fruit sugars. One reason for the power source of energy provided by raw fruit is the bulky residue produced by pectins, the alkalizing action of the fruit on the intestinal contents, and the slow release of the vitality-creating carbohydrates. Cooking will alter the energy-giving carbohydrates and render them less effective.

RAW FOODS HELP PROTEIN UTILIZATION. As a housewife, Stella W. was always too busy for proper eating. While she fed her husband and youngsters an adequate diet, she was always eating canned or processed foods or the so-called pre-cooked and convenience packages. She just "never had time" for herself. In due time, Stella developed a serious condition of low blood sugar, nervous temperament, and a chronic chill of her hands and feet. Her blood count was poor. Unable to stand in the kitchen for long hours, she avoided cooking by eating raw fruits and vegetables. In fact, one day, it was her entire fare. By nightfall, she felt invigorated and energetic. The raw fruits and vegetables had served to utilize protein that helped regulate Stella's blood sugar, nervous condition and the enrichment of her blood. It is hoped she will learn from Nature that raw foods are the foundation of good health.

How Raw Fruits Give a Protein Boost. The carbohydrates of raw fruits are not only highly digestible but also protein-boosting, an added asset. This action is maximally effective when protein and carbohydrates are ingested simultaneously. That is, when a main protein meal (meat, fish, eggs, cheese, beans, nuts) is finished with a raw fruit, the released carbohydrates help boost the health-building power of the protein. Furthermore, raw fruits are rich in dextrose, levulose and sucrose—simple and natural sugars that give a boost to the function of protein in the system.

RAW FOODS ARE TREASURE SOURCES OF ENZYMES. Raw fruits and vegetables are rich in enzymes, the substances that go to work on ingested food, take out the precious vitamins, minerals, proteins, carbohydrates and send them to the body's network for the purpose of building health. All raw foods contain enzymes; cooking will destroy these catalysts or life-forming agents. This means that you deprive your body of the necessary materials needed for repair and maintenance.

How Raw Foods Can Revitalize the Digestive System

The term "bad stomach" applied to nervous and edgy Barbara T. She felt stabbing pains whenever she ate the same food that neighbors appeared to enjoy with gusto. Barbara T. scoffed at eating raw fruits and vegetables. She said that she much preferred pre-cooked or canned foods because they had already been pre-digested by processing, thus sparing her "delicate condition" this painful procedure. But Barbara T. became chronically ill and was so weak and exhausted that she could scarcely go about her daily household chores. It was when a neighbor who came in to help insisted upon giving her fresh and uncooked foods, that Barbara T. began to recover. But no sooner did she attain the digestive power of a healthy person than she went back to the mushy cooked foods and now impaired her health to the level where she began to develop ulcer conditions. By this time, health restoration was a dim hope. Barbara T. had only herself to blame. Raw foods could have strengthened and nourished her digestive system and given her the rich enzymatic power she needed for overall health.

Raw Foods Aid Digestion. As ripening of raw fruits and vegetables proceeds, the activity of starch-splitting enzymes increases and raw food starch is converted into natural sugar. This quick change of texture and flavor is one reason why raw fruits and vegetables are like healers and natural boosters to the digestive system.

Raw Foods Stimulate Regularity. Janet W. was a schoolteacher with a problem. No, not the boisterous youngsters in her class; rather, irregularity. She was also addicted to the "laxative habit." It meant that she frequently had to excuse herself in the midst of a lesson to go to the bathroom. This was embarrassing as well as inconvenient. Furthermore, the laxatives weakened her system so that she became dependent upon them. How to stimulate and establish natural regularity? It came about one rainy day when she was unable to go to the adjoining building for lunch in the cafeteria. A teacher friend gave her several helpings of raw fruit. Janet W. ate them with gusto, and felt a pleasant digestive sensation.

The teacher friend said that fruit—raw and uncooked—was Nature's own regularity device. Janet W. wondered whether this was an intentional hint about her own frequent bathroom trips. She decided to give up laxatives. Nightly, she would eat a bowl of seasonal fruit. Mornings, with breakfast, a whole fresh apple, pear or banana. Throughout the day, she would finish her meal with more fresh fruit. Vegetables were always cooked. Result? She had partial and occasional regularity. Next step? Eat *raw* vegetables. Result? She had normal regularity and ended the laxative habit.

RAW FOODS HELP NORMALIZE DIGESTION. Most fresh, raw fruits and vegetables help to favorably change the number and variety of intestinal organisms. Fruit pectin sucks up bacteria which then are discharged. In constipation, it changes bacterial flora, adds bulk to intestinal contents. Raw fruit is also beneficial because it is easily assimilated, conserves protein, helps prevent formation of ketone acids (substances that may upset the delicate acid-alkaline balance of the system), and thereby reduces the quantities of urinary solutes. Raw foods may well be considered Nature's own digestive tonic.

How Raw Foods Can Improve Appetite

Raw foods can serve to revitalize and stimulate the appetite. It can also awaken the mouth and taste to the unique and delicious taste thrills of wholesome food. Here are some of the benefits of raw foods:

1. *Helps provide jaw exercise.* Raw foods require more chewing and therefore will supply the jaw and teeth with much needed exercise. This helps strengthen the jaw muscles.

2. *Starts natural flow of digestive juices.* Ralph Y. always gulped down his food. This constant bolting of half-chewed pre-cooked food and scalding beverages so ruined his digestion that his "stomach felt all tied up in knots" whenever he ate anything. Furthermore, Ralph Y. was getting dizzy spells, caught one allergic symptom after another, began to develop a stooped, bent-over condition. Arthritic tendencies showed in his stiff fingers and joints. Ralph Y. followed doctor's orders by getting more rest, easing tension, eating leisurely and eating uncooked foods. The program helped. Ralph Y.'s chewing of raw foods insured proper insalivation. Furthermore, the chewing process automatically called for a flow of digestive enzymes which served to attack the ingested food and extract necessary

healing nutrients. Ralph was on the way to recovery. Even his stiff fingers and joints became more flexible. But—growing overconfident and anxious to make up for lost time (he considered eating a waste of time), he went back to bolting down his pre-cooked foods and soon had to require hospitalization. He had bleeding ulcers and anemia. Now, recovery appeared to be doubtful and definitely prolonged. He had his chance but he tossed it away.

3. *Raw foods help restrict unnecessary seasoning.* The harsh action of volatile salt, pepper, artificial seasonings such as ketchup, mustard, biting vinegar, all tend to create a corrosive (burning) sensation in the delicate tissues and cells of the body. Furthermore, these artificial additives whip up the circulation and create blood pressure upheaval. To help resist the temptation to use harsh salt, pepper and other condiments, raw foods are beneficial. Raw vegetables have their own natural flavors that satisfy the taste buds of the mouth and tongue. Furthermore, when food is eaten raw, it cannot be overly seasoned since it would be "hot" upon tongue touch. But when food is cooked with harsh seasoning, the taste is dulled and the burning sensation is minimized, although it still has its vicious inner consequences. Raw fruits and vegetables serve to satisfy. the taste for sharp condiments.

4. *Raw foods are usually fresh.* There is life and health in fresh foods. Surely, a fresh raw apple is a greater source of skin-building Vitamin C than one that is cooked. A bowl of raw fresh vegetables is extremely rich in precious blood-building minerals, compared with pre-processed vegetables taken out of a can or bottle. Raw foods are precious sources of the life giving substances that provide abundantly healthful living.

5. *Raw foods are safe to eat.* Raw foods, even if spoiled, cannot be camouflaged and passed off as good food, as can cooked foods. When raw fruits or vegetables begin to spoil because of over ripening or other reasons, you can see it. But when the same raw food is pre-cooked, canned or bottled and later placed before you, then you have no way of knowing whether it was once live food—or dead food! So raw foods may

well be considered a form of health insurance. At least, you can see what you are eating!

Let Nature Do the Cooking of Food

Foods that have been ripened and brought to a state of maturity by Nature may be considered cooked by the natural forces of sunshine. Think of Nature-cooked foods such as a luscious bunch of purple grapes swinging to and fro in bowers of green.

Or of a hickory nut that has ripened in the top of a mountain tree, whose life-giving properties have been filtered through a hundred feet of clean, white wood.

Or of a delicious apple, or peach, reddened, ripened and finished—nursed in the lap of Nature, rocked in her ethereal cradle, and kissed from the fragrant blossoms of infancy on to maturity by the soft beams of the life-giving sun, ready for eating joy.

They are perfect. They are cooked by Nature. They are rich in the nourishing nutrients that give you life and precious health.

Eat Food That Is Born—not Made

Sylvia E. was a prosperous dress designer, working from her cozy home-studio. She had plenty of customers with whom she would chat while doing the fittings. Because Sylvia wanted to keep herself slim, to set a good example as should any fashion designer, she would eat modestly. She would avoid heavy, rich, creamy desserts as well as fatty foods. She would eat nourishing food such as fat-trimmed cuts of meat, fresh water fish, fruits, vegetables, cottage cheese, various beans and nuts. She never used sugar. Sylvia E. may have been slim—but she looked "under the weather."

Cooked Foods Sap Vitality. Sylvia E. may have eaten fruits and vegetables but they came from a can or bottle and were always pre-cooked or pre-processed. She denied herself the perishable vitamins, minerals, enzymes and natural carbohydrates that would provide healthful vitality.

Cooked Foods Upset Energy Balance. Frequently, Sylvia would feel her nerves on edge. She repressed the desire to snap at her customers. She felt nervous tremors, a throbbing of the temples and a heavy weight in the small of her back. There were times when she had to cancel appointments in order to lie down and try to take a nap while she was in a fitful frame of mind. She was nervous and temperamental. She later learned that the canned and bottled foods she ate were all soaked with white sugar, creating an upset in her blood sugar level which led to hypoglycemia, the reverse of diabetes. In other words, Sylvia had too little sugar in the bloodstream because she was deficient in vitamins, minerals and protein; the sugar in the processed foods was utilized at an alarmingly fast rate.

Cooked Foods Caused Complexion to Grow Sallow. This unhealthy and unnatural diet caused Sylvia's skin to become blotchy. She developed unsightly acne and bumps. The pink blush of youth gave way to a sallow complexion. Even the backs of her hands became blemished and yellowish. She became understandably upset over her condition.

RAW FOOD PLAN RESTORES NATURAL HEALTH

Sylvia might have gone down into health loss had not one of her customers noted her fading health and urged her to improve her living habits. When the customer was invited to have lunch with Sylvia, she saw the array of canned and bottled foods. She refused. She said that she wanted to eat *live* food—to enjoy her own life—and not dead food which would only hasten the aging process. The customer and Sylvia worked to prepare a simple, tasty and natural raw food eating program that helped restore the dress designer to the bloom of youth.

Here is the simple program:

BREAKFAST: Fresh raw fruit in season, with some cottage cheese and a slice of whole grain bread. A soft boiled egg; a whole grain cereal with unbleached raisins.

LUNCH: Raw seasonal vegetables with salad dressing; baked or broiled fish slice with side dish of raw vegetables such as radishes or lettuce or tomatoes. Dessert could be any seasonal fruit such as banana, apple, pear, berries, etc. The emphasis here is on *raw*, uncooked fruit.

DINNER: A big bowl of *raw* vegetables. Use natural salad dressing of desired oil with lemon juice for tang. Main dish could be fat-trimmed meat, poultry, fish or a meat-substitute dish, or a dish of cooked vegetables. (Yes—you may eat cooked vegetables since many cannot be consumed when raw.) Dessert could be a dish of seasonal fruit with a topping of honey.

DESIGNER'S HEALTH NOW RETURNS VIA RAW FOOD. Sylvia felt her health and appearance returning. The secret here is that the *raw* fruits and vegetables helped nourish her system with the perishable vitamins, minerals, enzymes, carbohydrates. She could eat cooked vegetables and even cooked fruits, but they had to be passed up in favor of raw foods. Furthermore, the preservatives and sweeteners used with pre-processed foods tend to upset the hormonal-sugar-endocrine balance which regulates the body's mind and health. Sylvia still partakes of processed foods but makes raw foods her prime concern.

The Vital Health Benefit—Eat Food That is Born—Not Made!

Fresh fruit of all kinds should be eaten raw. There are virtually no fruits that require cooking. Make it a rule of thumb to eat fruit *raw* as much as possible.

Fresh vegetables that *can* be eaten raw, should be eaten raw. For example, celery, cabbage, carrots, cucumbers, turnips, tomatoes, lettuce, onions, parsley, greens of all kinds, watercress, are just a few that should be eaten raw. They are brimming with digestion-helping enzymes, blood-building minerals, skin-tissue-cell-building vitamins. These succulent, juicy good vegetables are LIVING FOOD and will provide LIVING HEALTH to the body.

Other vegetables that can be cooked include beets, cauliflower, potatoes, kale, okra, parsnip, pumpkin, sweet potatoes, squash.

HOW TO COOK AND PRESERVE NUTRIENTS. When cooking vegetables in water, put them in boiling water, using just enough water to cook them done. Use leftover water for soups or broths. The vegetables should boil continuously after starting; if left to simmer for endless hours, they become water-soaked and lifeless, except for some bulk. You need not boil hard; just boil moderately.

RAW GRAINS ARE RICH IN B-COMPLEX VITAMINS. Richard F. is anxious to improve his nervous condition. He carries a little bag of whole grains (wheat germ, barley, oats, corn) and munches throughout the day. Now, Richard F. does have a nervous condition and he is extremely overweight. He knows that the Vitamin B-complex found in non-processed whole grains will not only help to feed the nervous system, but that one vitamin (B-6, or pyridoxine) is necessary to help the body assimilate essential fats. It is true that whole grains—raw and uncooked—will help Richard's nervous system and also help to assimilate the added fat.

But it is also true that Richard F. is abusing his health by eating processed foods, keeping late hours, rarely eating fresh raw foods, drinking caffeine-containing coffee and tea.

Richard F. is just deluding himself. He thinks there is just *one* way to restore health. He is trying to compromise with Nature and will only worsen his health if he discards the rest of Natural Laws for Abundantly Healthful Living.

THE ENTIRE HEALTH BUILDING PROGRAM PROVIDES MAXIMUM BENEFIT. It should be emphasized again that our bodies need, not single food elements by themselves, but a suitable assortment of all. When we say *all,* we mean *all.* If the health seeker eats some nourishing food, yet continues to spoil his body with improper living habits, he will lose the benefits of natural health. *Raw foods, for example, form the foundation for maximum health benefit.* Give your body the working materials with which to create living health and you have formed a solid foundation for inner rejuvenation and outer revitalization.

HIGHLIGHTS OF CHAPTER:

1. Raw fruits and vegetables are Nature's staff of life. They

are prime sources of vitamins, minerals, enzymes, carbo-hydrates, natural fats. These nutrients are depleted or evapo-rated in cooking.

2. Raw foods have nutrients to enrich the bloodstream, power up the energy system, assist in protein utilization.

3. For digestive problems, raw fruits help stabilize the enzymatic system and provide healthful regularity without laxatives.

4. Raw foods help improve appetite, provide jaw exercise, start natural flow of enzymatic juices for natural digestive power of a youngster; they also put a natural curb on the urge for excessive seasoning.

5. A health rule of thumb—EAT FOOD THAT IS BORN—NOT MADE.

6. Each day, eat raw fruits or vegetables; a small portion with each meal is healthful.

7. Raw food forms the foundation and is a basic law for healthful living. The "healing wellsprings" within your digestive system become fountains of youth when energized by nutrients released from raw foods. For your health's sake, *eat raw what can be eaten raw,* cook all foods that *must* be cooked.

3

FOODS TO EAT
FOR A MORE YOUTHFUL SKIN

Eleanor T. was dissatisfied with what she saw in her mirror. Although she was a trim 40-years-plus, she looked much older because her skin had furrows, creases, age spots. Eleanor T. was worried because she was in a local dramatic club production where youthful looks meant so very much. When the casting director said she ought to play the "grandma" role of the play, Eleanor T. flinched and held back her tears. That was when she decided to do something about her skin.

Hollywood Secret of "Skin Food"

It was from a well-known Hollywood actress, who was appearing in a local summer stock show at the same theatre, that Eleanor T. learned that the skin should be fed a certain everyday food, obtainable in every market. The actress suggested a Hollywood Skin Food to be applied nightly. The secret here is that this particular formula, made from three items found in every kitchen pantry, applies an acid mantle to the naturally acid skin; it also is a prime source of tissue-building protein which is the youth restoring nutrient of the body. Eleanor T. prepared this easy formula:

HOLLYWOOD SKIN FOOD. Mix one-half cup of mayonnaise with the beaten white of an egg. Add several drops of the beaten white of 1 egg, 1 tablespoon powdered milk, 2 tablespoons laundry starch (crush to powder, if lump starch), and 1½ ounces apple cider vinegar. Mix to form a light paste. cologne or perfume for pleasant scent. Use this Hollywood Skin Food as a night cream. Rub well into the skin with a gentle massage movement at night before retiring. The combination of protein (from mayonnaise) and natural acid forming ingredients (egg white) with the alcoholic astringent of the cologne exerts a soothing and nourishing effect upon the skin. It reportedly helps lessen lines, wrinkles and crow's feet and eases the lines around the mouth caused by the wearing of dentures. Benefits are noticeable if the Hollywood Skin Food is used nightly for about five weeks.

SKIN GLOWS WITH HEALTH. When Eleanor T. used this Hollywood Skin Food together with a daily diet of lots of fresh raw fruits and vegetables for internal cleansing, and got plenty of sleep, she felt a tightness and an exhilaration of the skin. It took close to four weeks before the healthful glow appeared. Now she was given a "daughter" role in the play. Nature had scored a hit!

How the Acid Mantle Nourishes Your Skin

Nature provided your skin with a pH (acid) mantle that will vary from 4.5 to 5.5. Your skin should be "acid-balanced." The same applies to your hair. Doctors have found that at a pH of 4.5, your hair has its greatest elasticity, strength and luster. Ideally, your hair, like your skin, should be maintained at this level for the bloom of youth and health.

As a matter of fact, the fabric industry regularly treats woolen fabric with pH liquids to enhance their luster, resilience and feel.

AN ALL-NATURAL SOURCE OF ACID. The white of an egg is a prime source of natural acid that is highly nourishing to the skin and hair. By using egg white (beaten) in the following all-natural kitchen-made lotions, you will help to restore and maintain your natural acidity. This protects your skin and hair from harmful bacteria that can cause irritation and lead to loss of youthful texture. For the following kitchen-made lotions, use the *beaten* white of an egg.

SKIN-AWAKENER FACIAL. Combine these kitchen items: Apply to face; let remain for 30 minutes, then remove with wash cloth and cool water. Benefit is that it helps give a natural acid to the face and helps awaken sluggish cells.

ELBOW-SOFT CREAM. When Phyllis W. heard others whisper behind her back that she ought to wear long sleeves because of her "alligator elbows," she went home and broke out in a crying spell. She started wearing long sleeved dresses until her sister-in-law asked about them and then the truth came out. The kindly relative told her that she used grandma's old-fashioned Elbow-Soft Cream. She even helped Phyllis prepare it as follows:

Mix ½ cup water with the beaten white of 1 egg. Blend well. Apply to dry, rough, scaly elbows. Rub in well, twice daily. Do it the first thing upon arising in the morning. Do it again before retiring. Do not rinse off. After the third morning, rinse before a new application, every single morning. Continue until the "alligator elbows" become peach soft.

Phyllis W. marvelled at this all-natural "grandma" healer when her elbows looked young and smooth. Now she could wear short sleeves again. She made Elbow-Soft Cream a regular ritual. Just minutes a day added up to lovely skin. The secret here is that the natural acid mantle had been restored to the chafed elbows.

The Natural Food That Nourishes a "Starved" Skin

Nature has graciously supplied your skin with a tough, resilient constitution in a set of five layers. The top layer, the *stratum corneum,* is made of insoluble and soluble protein, dialyzable material (mostly amino acids), totaling 85 percent protein, 7.9 percent lipid (fats and oil), and 5 percent cell membrane. The basic ingredient of the skin is *protein* and a natural oil that protects you from the ravages of sun, wind, smoke, smog, dirt. Protein is a natural food that can nourish a starved skin, to help feed it with necessary tissues, cells and membranes.

PROTEIN BUTTERMILK FACIAL. Soak ½ cup of rolled oats (quick cooking) in 1 cup of buttermilk (churned-type, not Bulgarian) overnight. Strain through cheesecloth. Now add the beaten white of 1 egg to the liquid. Apply to your face and neck generously with a man's shaving brush (available at any pharmacy or drug store). Let remain for 30 minutes. Remove with cool water and wash cloth.

Ice Rub for Skin Rejuvenation. After the preceding facial, you can help give a get-up-and-glow look to your skin with this ice rub. Put one ice cube in two layers of cheesecloth. Gently rub into the entire face, forehead and neck. The benefit here is that this two-step program helps to eliminate a "sallow" complexion, then invigorates the sluggish cells in the network right beneath the surface of the skin. If you follow this all-natural two-step program at least once daily for several weeks, the results will be astounding.

How Nature Builds Skin-Youth From Within

As a practicing certified accountant, Arnold Y. came in contact with a lot of people. His appearance could mean the difference between success and rejection. In fact, appearance is often more influential than ability, even though the person is qualified. But Arnold Y. was all business. He rightfully felt that his talent for auditing should stand on its own merit. But his blotchy skin, his crow's feet, his bumpy exterior gave the impression of sloppiness. This made him unwelcome at business meetings and he even lost some clients. Arnold Y. learned that for some clients, an appearance sells more than the work!

SKIN-YOUTH EATING PLAN. It was a doctor-client who noted Arnold's skin (the doctor was a dermatologist or skin specialist) and suggested the following tasty and healthful eating plan. The benefit here is that the Skin-Youth Eating Plan is low in fat but has goodly amounts of protein and moderate amounts of carbohydrates. Arnold Y. could have his taste buds satisfied while his skin received good amino acid nourishment. Here is the special eating plan:

Foods That Nourish the Skin

Skimmed milk
Fatless meats, boiled or broiled
Potatoes
Fruits and vegetables, all kinds, preferably raw
Margarine
Fresh fish (broiled)
Fruit juices, unsweetened
Eggs (poached or boiled)
Sweetening from a natural source such as honey

Foods to Avoid

Chocolate	Gooey desserts
Nuts	Pies and pastries
Pork	Fried foods
Bacon	Shellfish
Ham	Iodized salt
Cream	Cola and soft drinks
Greasy foods	Alcohol (all forms)
Homogenized milk	Sharp cheese
Butter	Dates
Hot Coffee	Sugar
Cocoa	

The Feeding of Arnold's New Youth-Skin. Nature decreed that healthy or youthful skin starts with proper inner health. Arnold derived a youth-skin appearance by following the preceding eating plan. Now he looked healthful and was no longer scowled at by others. But he became overly confident, started eating the taboo foods and neglected himself. He developed severe acne that was so deep he would have unsightly pits and scars. Now he required chemotherapy tnat offered partial relief. Arnold, like others sought to compromise with Nature. And, like others, he reaped what he sowed!

The Amazing Benefit of Baby Oil

A famous broadway actress, Lynne L., continues to play youthful roles to packed theatre audiences. Lynne L. is aware that her skin must look young because the strong stage floodlights expose any wrinkles or creases. Lynne L. learned that the most nourishing emollient for the skin is simple *baby oil*. She uses it to lubricate her skin, then to remove makeup, and, on occasions, she will refrain from washing and let a covering of baby oil anoint her skin from morning until night. The reward? She is as young as always!

How Baby Oil Can Give You Baby-Soft Skin. Since the oil is made for infants, it must be gentle and soothing. Baby oil is made of highly refined crude oil with removal of aromatic compounds which may cause irritation. Emulsifiers used in baby oil are very bland. Baby oil undergoes rigid testing for purity. This adds up to soothing skin softness for the skin.

The Magic Oil For Natural Skin Bloom

Research has discovered that in climates with higher humidity, less moisture is lost from the skin. This explains why the skin looks younger during a warm, humid summer than a dry, hot one. The English women who live in a moist, cool climate retain inner skin moisture and are rewarded with beautiful complexions. The secret here is to help *retain inner* skin moisture.

How to Keep Inner Oil. When the skin retains water, it develops a natural moisture that makes it look youthful with a healthful bloom. To help prevent the loss of precious inner oil and water, it has been found that *salad oil* can be an effective natural lubricant. Salad oil is more beneficial because it is an "edible fat" and thereby helps in the useful replenishment of the skin oils. Salad oil is more beneficial than petroleum preparations such as mineral oils which do not have that absorbent quality that is needed.

DERMA-DEAR SKIN OIL. To make a remarkable and all-natural oil that helps to retain the needed inner moisture,

you may easily prepare this homemade skin food: Mix ½ cup
salad oil with 2 beaten egg whites. Mix thoroughly. Apply to
the face as an oil and let remain as long as possible. At night,
wash off with cold water and a wash cloth. If you use soap, it
should be an acid-containing soap to maintain the pH or acid
mantle. Or, add juice of 1 lemon to rinse water to help restore
acid mantle.

Magic Benefit of Derma-Dear Skin Oil. The fatty acids of the
oil and the rich protein of the egg white both join to help
Nature stimulate the youthful freshness of the skin. When used
in a combination, Derma-Dear Skin Oil provides substitutionary
fluids to help stimulate the sluggish intercellular functions of
the skin. In this Magic Combination, the two ingredients
become isotonically pressurized to balance successfully with
natural fluids. These two ingredients further provide a stimulation and replenishment of the plasma colloids (skin water-
bearers) by hygroscopic attraction to the skin of moisture
always present in the atmosphere. This helps retain inner skin
moisture and preserve and replenish natural skin health. Derma-
Dear Skin Oil is far superior to any emollient cream because the
latter acts only on the surface. Derma-Dear Skin Oil—made right
in your own kitchen from ordinary pantry items—encourages
the skin to absorb body moisture to help it become naturally
moist and pliable. It is used by many theatrical women who
look young even though they are well past middle age. Nature
rewards with healthful youth.

Cucumber Juice for Age Spots

Skin blemishes often respond to a folk lotion made of just
two kitchen ingredients. Mix 1 teaspoon of glycerine to ½ cup
cucumber juice. Massage a little into the face at night after
washing. Massage into any age-spot region. It reportedly helps
lighten blemishes and soothe away premature age spots.

CLEOPATRA'S SKIN SECRET. Legend has it that the
lovely Cleopatra would prepare a special Desert Beauty Oil that
brought out the exquisite softness of the skin. Here is the basis
of how she had it made:

Desert Beauty Oil. Mix equal portions of olive oil and rubbing alcohol and apply to the skin. The alcohol gives the mixture a pleasant feel and spreads the oil in a thin layer, then evaporates. Start with a half-and-half mixture, then thin it with alcohol until the coating of oil it leaves on your skin is in no way noticeable or annoying. We all know of the legendary beauty of the ageless Cleopatra. Why not use this simple Desert Beauty Oil to help Nature make you become a beauty in your own time?

Magic Benefit of Desert Beauty Oil. The secret of this all-natural oil is that it has a microscopic layer to hold in the precious moisture. The two ingredients become absorbed without interfering with the skin's "breathing." They serve to soothe and nourish the *stratum corneum* or the outer layer of the skin. While Cleopatra may not have known the scientific workings of the Desert Beauty Oil, she certainly made good use of it in charming Mark Anthony!

Water—Nature's Skin Healer

How Ordinary Water Can Exercise Your Skin. In a world where youth commands attention, Benjamin E. felt prematurely old. His company hired many younger men and he feared being held back in favor of others. While he kept a healthful diet and used skin oils, he still had less-than-satisfactory skin appearance. It was at an exercise club that he learned that *the skin needs exercise* for a pep-up and tone-up, just as do muscles and joints. Here is how Benjamin E. was able to use water to heal skin blemishes and exercise the skin:

1. Wash the face in warm water that is gradually increased to become as hot as comfortably tolerated. Use a wash cloth and apply to the skin to provide a homemade steam pack. Continue for five minutes.

2. Now wash the face in cool water that is gradually made to become as cold as comfortably tolerated. Again, use a wash cloth and apply to the skin to provide a homemade *cold* steam pack. Continue for five minutes.

3. Now turn on both faucets and use hot water and then

cold water alternately to splash your face. Finish with a brisk tepid water rinse.

BENEFIT OF USING WATER TO EXERCISE THE SKIN.

Benjamin E. reaped these healing benefits of water-exercise: the warm water increased circulation, relaxed the temperature, pulse and respiration; it served to increase the porous action of the skin to perform perspiration and absorption. The *cold* water created instant contraction of the small arteries because of its influence on the sympathetic nervous system. It served to relax the blood flow at first, and then it resulted in a slight increase in the rate of pulsation. It is this *contrast* that performs an exercise for the skin.

Benjamin E. found his skin looking younger; but more important, he felt better and he could function with the vitality of a youth. While he did not get the coveted promotion which went instead to a younger man (his company placed undue emphasis upon calendar years rather than biological years), he was able to resign and join another firm for a higher position and a salary increase. He worked better because he looked and felt better. Skin exercising is now a daily ritual.

Massage Your Way to Firm Skin

Geraldine P. would slap on cosmetics in the hopes that they would disguise her sagging skin. While cosmetics do add to personal appearance, they serve as a disguise! When Geraldine washed away the makeup at night, she washed away her youth! Or, as her inconsiderate husband would remark, "There goes your lovely face down the drain." Perhaps he was inconsiderate but there are times when a blunt comment leads to action. This time, Geraldine would try to stimulate her own sluggish skin muscles to become firm.

Simple Skin Massage. Geraldine P. heeded the advice of a noted dermatologist who suggested that when she apply her skin lotion at night, she rub it gently into the skin. Using the five fingers of both hands, she was to self-massage in this manner:

Forehead: Begin at bridge of nose and massage gently with both hands in an outward motion. That is, your ten fingertips are poised at the bridge and you massage from this base toward your temples.

Eye Sockets: Use the ten fingers and massage the skin lotion around the entire eye socket, from the eyebrows down to below the eye. Use a circular motion.

Nose: Use forefingers and middle fingers, to massage *down* the nose, the front and sides included.

Mouth Area: Use all fingers to massage the upper lip and the underside of the lower lip in a circular motion.

Cheeks: Use all fingers to massage the cheeks, from the corners of the mouth, in an *upward* motion.

Chin: Use all fingers to massage from the underside of the lower lip in a downward motion to the bottom of the jaw line. This counteracts the tendency of the skin to sag.

Throat: Massage from the jaw line down to the shoulder blades. Massage in a downward motion, from one end of the throat to the other. A downward motion helps firm up the sagging muscles of this particular portion.

BENEFIT OF FACIAL MASSAGE. Geraldine did benefit to an appreciable level so that her skin was better looking than before. Facial massage benefits by promoting circulation and exercising the facial muscles. A powerful benefit in facial massage is that it propels the blood to greater activity. This serves to nourish the skin cells that reward the person with a glow of youth. Geraldine still uses lots of makeup but her skin looks better because of proper nourishment, natural creams and lotions, regular facial massage. Now, her face no longer "goes down the drain" with her washed-off makeup!

Wash Out Your Insides and Glow On Your Outsides

Fresh water or fresh raw fruit and vegetable juices are a "must" in helping to self-cleanse your system. A lovely skin is an inside job. When you are well-scrubbed on your inside, you are well-scrubbed on your outside. Liquids are an essential constituent of the tissue cells and of all body fluids, such as digestive juices, too.

Juices Provide Natural Internal Scrubbing. A clogged system causes outbreaks of skin blemishes and unsightly blotches. Fresh juices or sparkling clear water help provide internal self-scrubbing. Juices dissolve nutritive material in the course of digestion so that it can be absorbed into the blood, which carries it to various parts of the body to repair and remove skin-harmful wastes. Juices further keep all mucous membranes of the body soft and prevents friction of their surfaces. Fresh juices and water will aid in regulating a normal body temperature and will also assist in body processes. It all adds up to a healthy skin which, after all, is as healthy as your insides.

Summary of Face-Saving Highlights:

1. The natural acid mantle of the skin holds the magic secret of youth-bloom. The Hollywood Skin Food is reportedly successful in helping maintain youth-building acid mantle.

2. To stimulate sluggish skin cells, use the easy Skin-Awakener Facial.

3. To soften "alligator elbows" try the homemade Elbow-Soft Cream.

4. Foods that nourish the skin shoud be part of the skin-nourishing program.

5. Baby oil and other natural homemade applications give a lovely "skin you just love to touch" benefit.

6. Use water to exercise your skin and refresh with a glow of youth.

7. Massage is a time-tested home method for firming up facial muscles. Take a few minutes. Benefit with a "years-off" skin.

8. Water and fresh fruit or vegetable juices wash out your insides and provide a healthful outside glow of skin health.

4

HOW TO USE FOOD COMBINATIONS THAT HELP CREATE YOUTHFUL DIGESTIVE POWER

When meals are prepared, does it matter to your digestive health in which way they are combined? The turn-of-the-century menus of fat-laden roasts, thick gravy, butter-soaked potatoes, fried vegetables, thick pie slab and strong coffee—did they combine properly to create rewarding health? Or did they eventually cause gaseous overweight, painful ulcers, wrenching stomach pains, a score of different gall bladder, kidney and heart troubles? We can all admit that there are some meals that make us feel better than others. It is possible to regain and rebuild natural health by the proper combination of foods.

The foundation law of abundantly healthful living is this one: *what you eat is not as important as what you digest and assimilate.* This precious assimilation of nutrients is improved by healthful food combinations that offer the key to a youth-producing digestive system. Let us see how it can benefit your health.

How Healthful Combinations Can Benefit Your Health

1. *Helps Balance Acid-Alkaline Ratio.* By eating acids and starches at separate meals, the alkaline environment in the digestive system is permitted to flourish and wash the insides without a gush of burning acid.

2. *Helps Sweeten Sour Stomach.* Corrective combinations reportedly help ease the problem of improper fermentation that may cause sour stomach.

3. *Helps Regulate Weight Conditions.* Digested sugar turns into weight-gaining starch; this may be assimilated and utilized if conflicting foods do not dilute and impede this valuable function.

4. *Helps Regulate Fat Distribution.* Fats may become trapped in the digestive system and seep into the bloodstream if there is an excess of heavy protein food ingested at the same time. The sharp pain in the chest may be a protest of trapped fat. By wisely regulating combinations, fat can be assimilated and help keep down the cholesterol level.

5. *Helps Control Gastric Distress.* Corrective combinations ease problem of acid-causing eructations (gastic distress and belching) that trigger internal distress. Often, gastric distress is so unpleasant it causes throat irritation, mucous flow and a burning cough of the throat and nose. Healthfully combined meals control gaseous fermentation and ease gastric distress.

6. *Helps Keep the Body Free of Excess Toxic Wastes.* Improper combinations become decomposed in the digestive system and release toxic wastes such as carbonic acid gas, bacterial acids, ammonia, alcohol. In an effort to neutralize, isolate and eliminate these toxic poisons, the body is forced to draw upon its precious vital reserves. This causes a robbery of the much-needed vitamins, minerals, enzymes, proteins, essential fatty acids which should be helping to build health.

7. *Helps the Body Retain Its Health-Building Resources.* Nature provided your body with a treasure of health-building resources. But their depletion may result from improper food combining; that is, during gastro-intestinal decomposition, the accumulation of toxic wastes signals Nature for nutrients to "wash out" and "scrub away" the debris. This may cause a shortage of delicate reserves elsewhere in the body. This is a silent, continuous depletion of the vital reserves, until by its sapping influence, it brings the body below the line of safety. In effect, it causes a bankruptcy of the body's powers of repair

and restitution. Improper food combinations can drain out the vital reserves. By corrective and tasteful combinations, the reserves can be built up to create digestive youth power—the key to natural health.

Acid-Starch Combinations

Natural Law: Do not eat acid and starch (carbohydrate) foods at the same meal.

Harold R. boasted he had a cast-iron stomach. Indeed, it felt like cast iron after he stuffed himself with any haphazard combination that tasted good. Once, during a business luncheon he ate heavily of bleached white bread and butter and also a bowl of canned fruit. In addition, he had a fried steak dripping with fat, and buttery-mashed potatoes. He ate fruit while he ate his other foods. He was enjoying the taste, when all at once his face became red, his eyes bulged and then he began to tremble. Suddenly, a knife-like pain sliced into his middle and he felt alternate hot-cold sweats. He could not finish the meal and had to be taken back to the office to be treated by the company nurse. He was given medication and sent home to rest for several days. Harold R.'s cast-iron stomach felt "rusty."

To avoid future attacks, he consented to some slight but healthfully beneficial eating changes. He would avoid eating acid and starch foods at the same meal. Furthermore, he would follow the suggestions listed in this chapter on healthful food combinations. He was *not* deprived of his eating pleasure, but he was asked to eat foods in healthful combination. Now his cast-iron stomach functioned smoothly and without sudden attacks.

Harold R. had a problem with improper acid-starch combination. Acid inhibited the digestion of starch and drained off the enzymes of the pancreas and intestines. This solidified the starch and created internal fermentation and eventual distress. When acid-starch foods are eaten *separately*, the enzymes are able to bring about digestion without interference or conflict. Simple but healthfully rewarding!

Protein-Carbohydrate Combinations

Natural Law: Do not eat a highly concentrated protein and a concentrated carbohydrate at the same meal.

This suggests that you separate the eating of nuts, meat, eggs, cheese or other concentrated protein foods at the same meal with bread, cereals, potatoes, sweet fruit, cakes, etc.

The assimilation-digestion of carbohydrates (starches and sugars) and protein is so conflicting that when they are mixed in the system, they interfere with the digestion of each other.

An acid process (gastric digestion) and an alkaline process (salivary digestion) cannot successfully be performed simultaneously in the digestion tract. In fact, undigested carbohydrates in large amounts in the stomach absorb pepsin (an enzyme) and thus prevent the acid from entering into combination with the protein to increase necessary hydrochloric acid. It is also reported that in the presence of carbohydrate, protein digestion is delayed, or improperly assimilated if at all!

How Separating Beans and Meat Improved Helen's Indigestion. While Helen Y. ate healthfully, she erroneously believed that the familiar "beans and meat" combination was satisfactory. She did not know it was a possible cause of her chronic indigestion. In fact, she spent a big portion of her kitchen budget money on stomach powders, alkalizers, fizz tablets and aspirins. She continued her improper protein-carbohydrate combinations until her stomach distress was too much and she discussed it with a nutrition-conscious niece. Now she was aware of the value of proper food combining. Her niece used the chart found at the end of this chapter as a guideline for Helen's corrective combinations. It helped. Helen ate protein and carbohydrates at separate meals. Her digestion improved. She considered herself cured.

Then she returned to her habitually improper combinations and developed such weak digestive power that she had to obtain prescription medicines for relief. It is believed that she may have developed an irreversible stomach problem. Improper food combinations can certainly deplete health!

BENEFIT OF SEPARATING PROTEIN AND CARBO-

HYDRATES. When a starch food such as beans or bread is eaten, comparatively little hydrochloric acid is poured into the stomach. The enzyme secreted upon bread or some starch food is neutral. When a concentrated protein food such as meat is eaten at the same time, a stronger digestive enzyme floods the system. These two contrasting processes—protein-digestion and carbohydrate-digestion—do not go on simultaneously with healthful efficiency. The neutral carbohydrate-enzyme dilutes the effectiveness of the strong protein-enzyme. In fact, digestion may be so diluted that it causes upset and stomach churning. Furthermore, delayed digestion leads to fermentation and eventual gaseous distress.

Protein-Protein Combinations

Natural Law: Do not eat two concentrated protein foods at the same meal.

Someone should have told Ruth C. The burning sensations in her chest that made her wince at the slightest provocation was probably caused by the unhealthy combination of protein-protein at the same meal. But Ruth C. was stubborn. She maintained that if it tasted all right, it was safe. She would carry her after dinner mints with her wherever she went. At home she had bottled medicines that were costly, as irritating to take as her condition, and certainly spoiled whatever rightful enjoyment was due her from food. Ruth C. had so-called "heartburn." It was undoubtedly caused by her improper food combination; chiefly, a protein-protein combination.

How One Protein at a Meal Can Relieve Digestive Distress. Two protein foods of different characters and different compositions will call for different and often conflicting types of enzymes and digestive juices. These contrasting digestive juices have different strength and character; if they are poured into the system at the same time, they may cause acidosis which results in a burning sensation in the food tube (esophagus) which passes near the heart in its passage from stomach to throat.

By eating just *one* protein at a meal, you are calling forth one basic digestive enzyme which can work at digestion without being diluted, diverted or distressed. This helps relieve conditions leading to digestive upset. Ruth C. apparently thought it easier to reach for a bicarbonate than to look to Nature for stabilizing the digestive process by taking one protein at a meal.

Protein-Fat Combination

Natural Law: Do not eat a protein food with a fat food at the same meal.

The conflict here is that fat depresses the action of the gastric glands and inhibits the pouring out of the proper gastric enzyme that is needed for assimilation of protein. The presence of fats in the stomach diminishes the production of the valuable protein enzymes.

Corrective Combination Improves Digestive Power. Anthony E. refused to accept the fact that he was over 40 years old. In order to prove to others that he was young he would eat any combination of food, as did some of his adolescent sons at the table. But as soon as he finished his meal, Anthony E. complained of a heaviness in his chest, an uncomfortable lump in his stomach. It took a false alarm, an appendicitis scare, to alert him to proper food combinations.

Anthony E. could continue to eat with the gusto of a youngster but in proper combinations. By separating protein and fat foods to be eaten at different meals, he was able to enjoy his food—while eating it and after eating it! He also followed correct combinations in the categories outlined in this chapter and now he could enjoy his food even more than a youngster!

Benefit of Separating Protein and Fat Foods. The presence of fat lessens the amount of secretion that is poured into the stomach and further lowers the amount of protein-digesting pepsin and hydrochloric acid. It is reported that as much as 50 percent of the gastric tone may be reduced by this improper combination. It may last for two or more hours; hence, the prolonged feeling of stomach-heaviness after such a meal. A benefit in separating protein and fat is that the digestive tone is perked up without this conflicting influence. Furthermore, those foods containing normal fat within themselves (nut, cheese, milk) require longer time to digest than those protein foods with lesser fat (such as fish, eggs, peas). To put both of them together is to upset the natural healthful digestive process. You can revitalize and invigorate your digestive system by separating protein and fat.

How to Eat Your Protein-Fat Combo with Nature's Secret Digest-Aid. Nina E., a librarian who manages a household at the same time, finds that there are occasions when she cannot separate protein and fat. She has discovered Nature's Secret Digest-Aid. Here is the secret:

Raw, fresh green vegetables are prime sources of natural enzymes. Nina E. eats an abundance of these vegetables—*raw*—with a protein-fat meal. The benefit here is that the natural enzymes help counteract the inhibiting effect of fat so that the proteins ingested can be suitably ingested. Nina E. would enjoy better overall assimilation of amino acids *without* eating excess fat at the same time; but since she is always busy, the use of raw vegetables as Nature's Secret Digest-Acid can be most beneficial. Of course, one should never be too busy for health. The time to take care of your health is when you have it. But if you find yourself otherwise occupied, the raw vegetable practice is a valuable one. It is a partial compromise with Nature.

Protein-Sugar Combination

Natural Law: Sugar (commercial sugar, syrup, any artificial sweetener) inhibits the assimilation of protein and should be eliminated from the food program.

Sugar has an inhibiting effect upon the secretion of gastric juice and upon the naturally healthful motility of the stomach. Sugar certainly does "spoil the appetite" as we all remember. But sugar further hinders protein digestion.

How a Sugar-Free Program Rejuvenated Benjamin R. Here was a bus driver who loved his sugar. Hardly a meal was consumed without including sugar in the form of sweetener.

Benjamin never realized that his growing feeling of tiredness, his sagging skin, his stooped shoulders, his brittle hair and his chilled hands and feet could be traced to an excess sugar intake.

It was a physician who suggested he eliminate sugar. It was difficult for Benjamin R., who had a sweet tooth (to put it mildly), to give up his candy, cakes, syrups, confections, etc. But when he found his nerves getting on edge and his driving impaired, he had to do it.

In addition, he eliminated unnatural seasoning, ate many fresh raw fruits and vegetables, drank freshly squeezed juices, and set about to improve his health. It took four weeks before he looked and felt better. His posture was erect, his skin and hair improved, his hands and feet felt warm, his driving was perfect. Protein was now able to do its work in building the body. All that you see of yourself—and much of what you cannot see—is made of protein. But protein has to be assimilated in order to create the building blocks of your body. Sugar, when eaten with protein, is sent to the intestine for digestion. Often, sugar interferes with protein digestion to the level that it undergoes fermentation. This denies the body its rightful share of usable protein in the form of amino acid. Sugar can have that destructive effect. It had already done it to Benjamin R., who was wise to adjust in time.

To reap the reward of natural abundant living, it is wise to eliminate refined or artificial sugar from the New Diet. To please your sweet tooth, use honey, molasses, sweet herbs and sweet spices, carob powder, rose hips powder, date powder. Many of these all-natural sweeteners are sold at health food shops and super markets.

Sugar-Starch Combination

Natural Law: Sour stomach and acid indigestion are often traced to the eating of sugar-starch foods at the same time. Soothe your digestion by eating sugar (if you must!) and starch at separate meals.

Sugar does not undergo digestion in either the mouth or stomach, but rather, in the small intestine. When consumed alone, sugars are speedily sent out of the stomach into the intestine.

Starch digestion begins in the mouth and continues, under proper conditions, for a considerable length of time in the stomach.

When sugar and starch foods are consumed at the same time, they are held up in the stomach in order for other foods to be digested. While waiting, the combination of sugar-starch causes self-fermentation under conditions of warmth and moisture existing in the stomach. This leads to *acid fermentation.* Symptoms are felt as indigestion, sour stomach, belching: distress that calls for costly and distasteful medication.

Sugar with starch means fermentation and a sour stomach and discomfort. Perhaps baking soda, bicarbonate of soda, certain stomach salts, bile salts or fizz powders may neutralize the resulting acids, but the fermentation is still there. Surely, it is more healthful and soothing to avoid acid fermentation and general stomach acidity by eliminating sugar entirely—or at least by avoiding taking it with a starch food!

Starch-Starch Combination

Natural Law: There may be only one kind of starch, but starchy foods differ greatly so eat only ONE starch food at a meal.

If two or more starch foods are eaten at the same time, one or the other is selected for digestion and assimilation and the other must wait its turn in the stomach; it may find its way into the digestive system and retard the digestion of other foods. This leads to fermentation, sour stomach and a general-feeling of reduced or impaired health.

As stated above as part of the Natural Law: there may be only one kind of a starch, but each starch food is different and requires slightly different digestion. To take one starch food at a time is to help avoid fermentation and to further permit the enzymatic system to digest the starch and send its byproducts to the storage depots of the body to await use in the form of energy, mental stamina and vital youth.

Milk: A Food by Itself

Natural Law: Milk is the food of the young and is not a required food for adulthood. But if milk is consumed, it is healthful if considered a food by itself, and taken by itself.

Sandra E. helped her husband in their general store. She frequently had to make a quick snack because customers kept coming in from morning until night. While business was good in their Wisconsin town, it could have interfered with their health.

Sandra E. liked milk and would drink two glasses with just about every meal. She often complained of a feeling of weakness in the ankles, hot flushes, blurred vision and a general letdown in health. No doubt her improper eating was one contributing cause; but it was her constant drinking of milk with her meals that caused her general ill health.

When a customer noticed it and suggested that she drink milk alone and not in combination, Sandra E. scoffed. So did her husband who refused to believe that there was anything wrong with either of them. He, too, had general ill health and malaise. But Sandra's husband tried the separate milk health law in secret and he soon bounced back to better health. He served as a good example to Sandra who followed suit with the same separation of milk from other foods.

Of course, this simple adjustment improved their health but they experienced frequent letdowns because their meals were usually pre-cooked or "instant" varieties. Perhaps Sandra or her husband will have to experience a complete collapse to become alerted to the benefits of natural foods. Some folks need a disaster to discover the simple truths of Nature.

Benefit of a Milk-by-Itself Program: The entire digestive-assimilation system is rejuvenated by following a natural program and drinking milk by itself.

Milk has a protein and fat (cream) content which makes it a poor combination with most foods. The first thing that occurs when milk enters the stomach is that it coagulates (forms curds). These curds tend to form around the particles of other foods in the stomach, thus insulating them against enzyme juices necessary for proper digestion. This prevents digestion-assimilation of other foods until after the milk curd is digested, which leads to fermentation and impaired digestion as well.

Milk Can Be Soothing. Milk acts as a gastric insulator and can be soothing when taken alone. Its cream inhibits the outpouring of gastric juices for some time. Milk does not necessarily digest in the stomach, but in the duodenum (the 8-to 10-inch length of the alimentary canal of the digestive system that follows immediately after the stomach proper); therefore, in the presence of milk, the stomach does not respond with its secretion. This can be soothing.

But if other foods are introduced along with the milk, it causes impaired, delayed malfunction of the digestion. It would be healthful and Nature-compatible to take milk alone, if it is to be taken at all.

The Youth Food That Is Nature's Magic Miracle

While there is no one single food that can exert a complete digestive rejuvenation, there is one youth food that can rightly be called Nature's Magic Miracle. That food is found in every produce market or supermarket—that food is the apple.

How the Apple Can Turn Back The Age Clock

Many of the so-called health problems of advancing age can be corrected by natural health laws; the delicious, juicy apple, as Nature's Magic Miracle, can help turn back the age clock by providing the following benefits:

The Apple Can Correct Constipation—the Natural Way. Pectin, found in a whole apple, is the substance that makes a fruit juice jell. Pectin is valuable to the intestinal tract. As the chief source of bulk in the intestinal contents, pectin, with its ability to take up a large amount of water, forms a mass that stimulates essential intestinal activity with soothing action upon the mucous membrane lining. (Laxatives create harsh injury to this lining.)

The Apple Can Improve Digestive Power. It is reported that meats served with fruit are more readily digested than meats alone. Salmon with lemon juice, turkey with cranberries, fish or fowl or meat with some fruit means overall better digestion. The apple sparks a natural hydrochloric acid secretion in the digestive system to help make meat more assimilated. This is beneficial because the apple promotes the digestion of protein; it induces conditions favorable to the absorption of iron and calcium, two minerals which enrich the bloodstream and strengthen the bones and nerves.

The Apple Can Detoxify the System. Rich in its natural minerals and water, the apple offers a good way to regulate body heat; it is a good source of vitamins and pectin which help detoxify the system and combat body poisons.

The Apple Strengthens the Mouth. Since all food comes through the mouth, it is an inviolate natural law for the mouth to be healthy. The apple is rich in vitamins and minerals that detoxify the mouth and nullify potentially harmful bacteria that may contaminate food that is eaten. Further, its supply of Vitamin C helps nourish the cells and tissues of the mouth, tongue and gums, and thereby provides natural resistance to infectious poisons.

Your Everyday Food Classification Chart

PROTEIN

Nuts (most)

All cereals

Dry beans

Dry peas

Peanuts

All flesh foods (except fat)

Cheese

Olives

Avocados

Milk (low protein)

STARCHES

(Carbohydrates are starches and sugars. I have separated them into three groups: starches, sugars and syrups, and sweet fruits.)

STARCHES: (Mildly Starchy)

All cereals   Cauliflower
Dry beans (except soy beans)   Beets
Dry peas   Carrots
Potatoes (all kinds)   Rutabaga
Chestnuts   Salsify
Peanuts
Hubbard squash
Banana squash
Pumpkin
Jerusalem artichokes

SUGARS AND SYRUPS

Brown sugar   White sugar
Milk sugar   Cane syrup
Maple syrup   Honey

SWEET FRUITS

Banana   Date
Fig   Raisin
Thompson & muscat grape   Prune
Sun dried pear   Persimmon

FATS

(The fats are usually all the fats and oils, as follows:)

Olive oil   Butter   Most nuts
Soy oil   Cream   Fat meats
Sunflower seed oil   Nut oils   Lard
Sesame oil   Butter substitutes Cottonseed oil
Corn oil   Pecans   Tallow
                     Avocados

ACID FRUITS

Orange   Tomato   Sour grape
Grapefruit   Lemon   Sour peach
Pineapple   Lime   Sour plum
Pomegranate   Sour apple

SUB-ACID FRUITS

Fresh fig	Sweet peach	Huckleberry
Pear	Sweet apple	Mango
Sweet cherry	Apricot	Nectarine
Papaya	Sweet plum	Quince

NON-STARCH AND GREEN VEGETABLES

(Here are the succulent vegetables which are starch-free and rich in digestion-boosting enzymes:)

Lettuce	Cowslip	Parsley
Celery	Chinese cabbage	Rhubarb
Endive (French)	Chive	Watercress
Chicory	Chicory	Onions
Cabbage	Mustard	Scallions
Cauliflower	Dock (sour)	Leeks
Broccoli	Turnip	Garlic
Brussels sprouts	Kale	Zucchini
Collards	Mullein	Escarole
Dandelion	Rape	Cardoon
Beet tops (greens)	Green corn	Bamboo sprouts
Turnip tops (greens)	Eggplant	Broccoli-de-rappe
Chard	Green beans	Summer squash
Okra	Cucumber	Asparagus
	Kohlrabi	Radish
	Sorrel	Sweet pepper

NATURE HAS A BUILT-IN PROTECTIVE DEVICE FOR NATURAL COMBINATION. To a single item of food that is a natural combination, the body can adjust its digestive enzymes, both as to strength and timing, to the eventual assimilation of the item. Nature has this built-in protective device in most foods. But when *two foods* are eaten with different, even opposite, digestive needs, this all-natural precise adaptation to digestion becomes difficult. It is imcompatible with the digestive system to abuse it with conflicting foods. Ally yourself with Nature and corrective food combinations for internal rejuvenation. Your health is built upon the foundation of *proper assimilation* through corrective combining.

Highlights of Chapter 4:

1. What you eat is not as essential as what you assimilate. Improve your digestive power with healthful food combinations.

2. Note the seven benefits for the proper combination of food.

3. Corrective food combining can help digestion, strengthen assimilation powers, relieve internal distress, tone up system.

4. A sugar-free program can revitalize the digestive system.

5. Milk, if consumed, should be taken alone.

6. The apple is Nature's Magic Miracle Food. It offers four basic youth-building benefits.

7. In building the Food Combination Program into your health quest, remember: *what Nature combines, Nature can digest. What man combines, man often finds indigestible.*

5

HOW TO USE ENZYMES TO SLOW DOWN AGING PROCESSES

There are close to 700 self-rejuvenation fountains within the body that have been placed there by Nature to help slow down the aging processes. In some reported situations, these built-in fountains have reversed the aging process and helped create a youthful vitality. These miracle fountains are known as *enzymes.*

HOW ENZYMES HELP BOOST SELF-REJUVENATION. Specifically an enzyme is a physiological catalyst. That is, it brings about a certain reaction without becoming part of that particular reaction. For example, the pepsin enzyme converts protein into skin and tissue-building amino acids to nourish the entire body. But pepsin, itself, does not become part of the skin. It remains in the digestive system, ready to create building blocks of youth from ingested food. Without these precious enzymes, food could not digest and the body would die!

It has been noted by many physicians that as the body grows older, its enzyme supply decreases and also weakens in its valuable youth-building properties. The key, therefore, to regaining and retaining youthful health may well be in the enzyme.

THE ALL-NATURAL SOURCE OF YOUTH-BUILDING ENZYMES. These precious substances are found in *raw foods.* This is the foundation for abundantly healthful living, as we have seen. Raw foods are rich sources of perishable enzymes. Plant foods are endowed by Nature to manufacture these soluble catalytic substances, colloidal in substance, powerful to split up ingested foodstuffs, take out youth-building vitamins, minerals, amino acids, carbohydrates, hormonal ingredients and other life-giving nourishment for the body and mind.

ENZYMES OFFER HOPE FOR YOUTH PROLONGATION. Since each enzyme is specific (that is, it acts upon only one class of food substance), it offers specialized hope for youth prolongation. For example, there is one enzyme that will act upon Vitamin A for better eyesight and skin and fat utilization; this enzyme cannot act upon other nutrients. There is another enzyme that works to extract and convert and assimilate Vitamin C to nourish the cellular structure of the body and build firm skin and tissue; it will not work on other nutrients. There are still more specific individual enzymes that will work upon the disaccharides (complex sugars), the amino acids, the blood-building nutrients. All work together to help create a youthful and healthful condition. All are valuable in reaping the benefits of the natural laws for abundantly healthful living.

HOW ENZYMES HELPED STOP THE AGING CLOCK FOR ANNA R. Here was a vital woman who succumbed to a very serious virus in the middle of a heavy snowstorm winter. Anna R. had such a sore throat, she could barely swallow any food. This led to her drinking lots of hot liquids, soups, broths, gruels, pureed foods. Eventually she recovered, but by now she had been so devitalized by cooked foods that she looked and felt very weak.

Anna R. continued on her cooked food program, hoping this would build her resistance to further winter distress. In fact, she became so habituated to cooked foods, she continued right on even after the winter was past.

Lack of Enzymes Begins to Age Her Because of Exclusive Cooked Food Diet. She began to wither away. Her skin looked wrinkled, her hair was stringy, her once lovely figure began to sag and her muscles made her look sacky. Her body processes began to wear out. Even her eyes had that aged lack-luster dullness. Now Anna R. was worried. She thought that the winter virus had created some permanent inner infection that was sapping away her life's vitality. The withering process was actually caused by a depletion of her vital enzymes. The cooked food diet was totally without these life-building substances.

How Raw Foods Help Stop the Aging Clock. She tried a change in her food plan. She now would eat raw what could be eaten raw, cook what must be cooked. Two weeks and there was a slight change. She continued the program of raw fruits and vegetables, raw seeds and nuts, fresh salads and non-processed cheese, and now the Aging Clock began to slow. After one month of this program, her skin became firm and had a youthful bloom, her muscles grew taut, her nerves were stable, her energy was revitalized. The raw food program was brimming with youth-building enzymes. It took two months until Anna R. was healthy again. Now she not only felt young, she looked young as well.

Anna R.'s Simple Enzyme Youth Program. Anna R. would begin each of her three daily meals with a large bowl of fresh raw seasonal fruits or vegetables. Her main meal of either meat, fish or eggs would, of course, be cooked. But all else had to be raw and non-processed. In this simple manner, she provided her system with the precious youth-building enzymes that helped stop the Aging Clock.

Where to Find the All-Natural Source of Enzymes

Fruits And Vegetable: These should be fresh and raw and uncooked.

Sweetening: Sugar of all types (even raw sugar) has *no* enzymes. Honey, if unheated during extraction, has precious enzymes.

Dairy: Raw milk is rich in enzymes. Pasteurized or homogenized milk has *no* enzymes. Processed cheese and pasteurized butter have been robbed of their enzymes. If you can obtain natural and non-processed dairy products from a local health store or produce outlet, you will be feeding yourself healthful dairy enzymes.

Processed Foods: Enzymes can be retained if foods are dried at mild temperatures. Thus, naturally dried fruits, spray-method dried raw milk, seeds and grains can all be a good source of enzymes.

Raw Grains: It is encouraging that research has indicated a greater enzyme source in uncooked grains than in raw vegetables. The enzyme power in sprouted grains is phenomenal. Grains are a "must" in the enzyme source that will help slow down the Aging Clock.

Frozen Foods: While the first choice should always be fresh and living food that is *born* and not made, there are circumstances or situations calling for prepared foods. While heat destroys enzymes in food, they can survive freezing. So while canned foods and canned juices have practically no enzymes, frozen foods *(if not first processed with heat)* do have enzymes.

How Chewing Can Supercharge Enzyme Power

Young Edward K. found himself falling asleep at the wheel when driving. To add to his distress, he was unable to concentrate on essential business matters that came up during important office conferences. He began to make mistakes. When he erroneously undercharged a customer and caused his company a serious loss, he was dismissed. Now he had to do something about his declining health.

Raw Food Enzymes Offer Partial Help. In remaking and rebuilding his health, he used natural foods as part of his program. With adequate exercise, rest, utilization of proper breathing, water, sunshine, he was able to bounce back—but it was a small bounce. Even though he would eat copiously of fresh raw fruits and vegetables, he still found himself sluggish and filled with inertia. He still kept dozing off and making mistakes. His nervous system was still irritated upon the slightest provocation. What was his problem? He gulped down his food. He short-changed himself, as he had his company, with improper preparation. Raw food enzymes can be released through proper chewing!

Enzyme Power Begins with Chewing. Mouth enzymes begin

the digestion of food. Chewing breaks up the food into smaller particles. Mouth juices, normally alkaline, contain an enzyme called *ptyalin* which acts upon starch, breaking this down into *maltose,* a complex sugar, which is further acted upon in the intestine by *maltase* and converted into the simple energy-building sugar *dextrose.* To bolt down food as did Edward K. is to render it partially insoluble. The enzymes in the raw foods are thus "locked in" and cannot be released to perform their health and energy providing functions. To stimulate digestive enzyme flow, chewing causes an outpouring in the digestive tract that will serve to assimilate body nutrients. The key to enzyme power is in chewing!

Edward K. was unemployed for a long time. This gave him enough time to eat so he began to chew his food thoroughly. In a short while, he felt better, performed better and was able to land a good job. It is hoped he will continue the natural process of adequate chewing to release the store of locked-in enzymes for overall health.

Your Enzyme Elixir Cocktail

Ella O. may have many calendar years behind her, but she has the appearance, vitality and wit of a young woman. Perhaps she has learned, the hard way, from the experience of her late husband. Oscar O. was a voracious eater of processed foods. He stuffed himself with heavy sweet and fatty foods. (In fact, so did Ella O.) Literally, Oscar ate himself to death at a young 48.

Ella Discovers Enzyme Health in Raw Foods. Ella, herself, declined in health. Overweight, chronic cold-catching, looking older than her years, she was determined to do something about it. As a widowed mother of two, she had to go to work but she was not as robust as someone younger. She found a time-consuming job which was strangely fortunate. It meant she had to cut down her prolonged cooking time to get the meals prepared. She relied heavily on raw foods. Each meal had a garden variety of fresh fruits and vegetables. This was economical, too. She would frequently utilize raw salads to become main meals. Her health bloomed as did that of her children.

Now she discovered how Nature's living juices—enzymes—could actually revitalize the body.

The Enzyme Elixir Cocktail. To help fortify herself and her youngsters, Ella O. prepared the following all-natural morning booster:

> ¼ cup apricot juice
> ¼ cup fresh orange juice
> ¼ cup pineapple juice
> 2 tablespoons papaya juice
> 2 tablespoons natural honey

Vigorously blend all ingredients together. Drink at once. It is especially enzyme-stimulating to drink early in the morning, before breakfast.

This Enzyme Elixir Cocktail is a powerhouse of natural food enzymes; furthermore, it serves to stimulate the flow of the body's own enzymes that help to digest and assimilate the precious youth-building nutrients.

How Enzymes Restored Youth

In a reported case history[1] a physician divided test animals into two groups. The first group was fed raw foods and reportedly remained healthy. The second group was fed exclusively on cooked food and milk that was pasteurized, evaporated, or sweetened condensed milk.

Enzyme Starvation Causes Aging. Without precious enzymes found in raw foods, the second group developed such reported problems as gingivitis, loss of teeth, loss of fertility, difficulty in child labor, irritability, diminished or warped physical responses, allergies, infections, diarrhea, pneumonia, heart trouble, kidney disease, thyroid disease, paralysis, etc.

How Enzymes Restored Youthful Health. When the physician gave this second group a program of natural and raw food, he reported that youthful regeneration began to take place. Of course, if the degeneration had progressed too far, there was only a partial turn back to youthful health. Enzymes hold the power of life, health and youth!

---

1. *American Journal of Orthodontics and Oral Surgery,* case history reported by Francis F. Pottenger, Jr., M.D..

How Enzymes Can Stimulate Heart Health

Vitamin E has long been known to benefit and normalize heart function. Yet processing depletes and destroys this valuable vitamin, normally found in whole grain foods, including whole grain cereals. At the same time, whole grain foods are prime sources of *phosphatase,* an enzyme that serves to spark the action of Vitamin E and also to help the body assimilate minerals. Enzymes can help improve heart health.

Enzymes in Whole Grain Cereals. The enzyme, phosphatase, is found in heart-helping abundance in natural, non-processed whole grain cereals, together with Vitamin E. When you eat a bowl of such whole grain cereal, digestion utilizes Vitamin E to help nourish the arterioles and valves surrounding and entwined with the heart. Phosphatase provides the power to utilize this necessary heart health vitamin. Cereal germ and bran (non-processed and natural) are top notch sources of phosphatase and Vitamin E. These foods are available at most health food stores and at many large food outlets.

Enzymes Are Destroyed by Cooking. Heat above 120° F. kills these living elements. Of all the known food elements, enzymes are the only ones that are known to be destroyed when foods are heated on the stove.

Cooked Foods Require Stronger Enzyme Action. Sophie K. loved mushy vegetables. She was also addicted to cooked fruit desserts. Now, there is little harm in satisfying the taste urge with cooked vegetables and fruit. But Sophie K. developed such a passion for cooked foods that she would not touch any fruit or vegetable in its raw, enzyme-rich state. While Sophie K. did not look ill, she felt distinct health depletion.

Enzyme Starvation Causes Health Decline. Sophie caught more frequent sniffling colds that lasted longer. She developed skin blotches and age spots that failed to respond to costly medicated skin creams. (A healthy skin is an *inside* job, remember?) Sophie found it difficult to bounce out of bed in the morning. She yawned a lot. Her arms and legs felt heavy. Her shoulders slumped. Plainly she was enzyme-starved. Further, she shrugged off the other natural health laws of fresh air, proper sleep, proper food combinations, natural foods and occasional controlled fasting. Sophie was aging on the inside. She would soon age on the outside. She was enzyme-starving herself with cooked foods.

Fainting Spells Bring Return to Nature. When Sophie developed frightening fainting spells, she decided to do something. With the help of her family doctor, she improved her basic living habits. She started eating more raw fruits and vegetables. She found it difficult because habitual tastes are hard to change, but she had to do it to regain her health. She used the following natural law as her basic enzyme-restoration program:

1. *Eat raw food that can be eaten as raw food.*
2. *Eat cooked foods that must be cooked.*

Enzymes Bring About Partial Rejuvenation. In a two-month span, Sophie felt revitalized and rejuvenated. But she still turned up her nose at raw fruits and vegetables; she ate them in moderation. Furthermore, she disliked whole grains and had to force herself to eat them. This meant that her health restoration was partial. Let up hope that Sophie will look to complete enzyme rejuvenation for more complete health restoration. Compromise with Nature and you receive a compromise in benefits!

HEALTH BENEFITS OF ENZYMES. In brief, enzymes can perform these valuable health benefits:

1. Enzymes will improve digestive power.

2. Enzymes will help regulate the hormonal system. They serve to regulate the outpouring of glandular products. These hormones regulate the growth, health, well-being and emotional stability of the individual. In illness, the body becomes corpulent or thin because of the malfunctioning of enzymes in the hormonal network of the body.

3. Enzymes exert a self-cleansing stimulus. By means of *autolysis* (self-loosening), enzymes help wash and scrub away internal debris and waste.

4. Enzymes often alleviate conditions of diabetes. One known enzyme is *secretin,* which activates the production of in-

sulin by the pancreas. This enzyme assists in sugar metabolism; overabundance of sugar may cause diabetes.

5. Healing processes are facilitated by enzymes. These miracle workers serve to extract vitamins, minerals and amino acids from food to use as building blocks that will serve to heal the body from everyday and more serious injuries.

Your Magic Enzyme Cocktail

Liquefy together 1/3 cup alfalfa seed and 4 cups water.

The seeds may be soaked for a while before liquefying, as they will liquefy easier when soaked; soaking for 30 minutes is sufficient. After liquefying, strain through a fine cloth. Squeeze to get out all the milk. (A clean flour bag may be used for straining seed milks.) Drink this milk as soon as possible. It is a powerhouse of raw enzymes that serve to exert a "magic" rejuvenation in the body.

You may keep this milk in the refrigerator, if you wish, but it is best to drink it as soon as possible. It is also a prime source of vitamins, minerals and blood-building protein as well as the dynamic infection-fighting enzymes.

Important Enzyme Facts in Review:

1. Enzymes are wonder workers that boost self-rejuvenation in the body and the mind.

2. The magic power of enzymes is in their natural ability to take out vitamins, minerals, proteins, amino acids and other nutrients from foods to help the body maintain and improve health. Without enzymes, food would just lie in the stomach in an undigested lump. The organism withers and may perish.

3. Enzymes are found in raw and non-processed foods such as fresh fruits and vegetables.

4. Chewing causes activity of the body's supply of enzymes to create greater digestive powers of nutrient-assimilation.

5. The Enzyme Elixir Cocktail, prepared with five natural ingredients found in any food store, can work wonders in health benefits.

6. Enzymes benefit and normalize heart action.

7. The Magic Enzyme Cocktail provides a power house of precious youth-giving enzymes. Just two ingredients (one is plain water) can create a "magic" rejuvenation to stop — and turn back — the Aging Clock. In truth, *You are as young as your enzymes!*

6

HOW TO GENERATE MORE BRAIN POWER EATING SELECTED FOODS

Daniel E. was starting to show signs of forgetfulness. He would neglect writing down pertinent information in his job as a wholesaler of farm machinery products. Daniel E. would often confuse names of lifelong friends, much to their mutual embarrassment. His hands would shake when he had to add several columns of numbers. Daniel E. even looked senile because of his blank expression when he was spoken to. His wife was upset over his inability to correlate events of the day. She was told that Daniel E. was losing his mind even though he was hardly in his early 50's. She hoped Daniel would get over this memory lapse and fumbling attitude, but she soon found he was getting worse. When the morning came that he just remained in bed, looking blank, she decided to call the family physician.

HOW CORRECTIVE FOOD RESTORED MENTAL YOUTH

The physician subjected Daniel E. to a battery of tests; chief among them was one to pinpoint his nutritional habits. Now the culprit was revealed. Faulty diet was basically responsible for Danies E.'s so called senility. Basically, *hypoglycemia* (or low blood sugar in which there is a deficiency of sugar supply in the system) was the fault. A special program of corrective foods was outlined for Daniel E. It worked wonders. It saved him from the dreaded "home for the senile" and it made him younger than ever before.

Here is the program that was outlined:

FOODS ALLOWED IN UNLIMITED QUANTITIES

DAIRY: All dairy products, including milk, buttermilk, cream, cheeses, eggs, butter.

MEATS: All forms of meats, prepared any style. *But*—no breaded cutlets, no breaded chops, no gravies thickened with flour, no stews with potatoes or rice.

FISH: All forms of fresh fish.

POULTRY: All forms of freshly prepared poultry.

NUTS: All kinds allowed, *except* peanuts, cashew, chestnuts.

Vegetables to Boost Mental Energy

green pepper	kale	asparagus
radishes	tomatoes	string beans
pumpkin	lettuce	wax beans
carrots	olives	Brussels sprouts
onions (cooked)	fresh peas	cabbage
squash	eggplant	celery
turnips	endive	spinach
	watercress	cauliflower
	broccoli	beets

Fruits to Boost Mental Energy

oranges	watermelon	blueberries
grapefruit	apples (peeled)	blackberries
lemons	pears (peeled)	raspberries
limes	peaches (peeled)	grapes
honeydew	pineapples	cherries
cantaloupe	strawberries	fresh plums (peeled)

How to Take Your Fruits: Take only *one* portion of fruit at a meal. That is, do not eat more than one orange or apple at a time. Applesauce prepared without sugar is suitable; apples may be baked *without* sugar. Do *not* use dried fruits.

BENEFITS OF THIS MIND-BUILDING PROGRAM. The magic benefit here is that this particular diet is high in protein but low in carbohydrates. It is reported that carbohydrate-rich foods have a depressant effect on bodily oxygen consumption because they reduce the delivery of glucose to the brain tissues for utilization. In situations such as those of Daniel E., the reduced glucose delivery to brain tissues results in a reduced glucose-oxygen consumption. This resultant asphyxia may further lower the resistance to bacterial invasion. The preceding food program provides a rich store of oxygen sent to the brain for its best functioning.

HOW THIS FOOD PROGRAM FEEDS YOUR BRAIN. Just like other body cells, you brain cells need oxygen and food. The blood carries these to the brain through four arteries. An insufficient supply of oxygen means the brain cannot adequately function. The food of the brain is basically blood sugar which is supplied by the goods described above; without this necessary "brain food" the level of sugar and oxygen in the blood becomes unbalanced. Hence, symptoms of so-called senility, or feeble-mindedness.

Foods to Avoid in a Mind-Nourishing Program

Avoid sugar, potatoes, corn, rice, barley, lentils, hominy, split peas, bananas, tapioca, macaroni, pancakes, noodles, spaghetti, cake, candy, pastries, malted milks, prunes, raisins, canned fruit juices, cereals, bread, rolls, toast, ice cream,

How Elimination of Above Foods Can Help Strengthen Brain Function. In situations where mental strength is needed, elimination of the above-listed foods can help regulate and normalize the supply of glucose in the system. The preceding "avoid" foods have a high sugar and starch supply which may lead to over-metabolization or "burning" of needed blood sugar. This causes depletion and also a shortage of necessary internally-created sugar. The blood is unable to supply the brain with necessary energy-creating sugar and there are symptoms of mental distress or senility. Elimination of these foods means that now there is an ample supply of blood sugar available for the body. Basically, it is a high-protein and low-carbohydrate food program that helps nourish the brain.

Build Other Natural Laws in Your Mind-Building Program. In order to help regain and retain mental and physical health, include the natural laws of proper rest, healthful exercise, natural foods. a large abundance of fresh, raw and succulent fruits and vegetables daily, occasional fasting to flush out internal wastes, and a general alliance with Nature. Obey the natural laws of Nature and be rewarded with vitalic living and health.

What You Eat Today—Thinks Tomorrow

Joan W. became nervous, edgy and temperamental. This unusual behavior disturbed the rest of her family. Even the women at the weekly club meetings she attended would avoid Joan because she was unreasonable, irritable and would snap at others upon the slightest provocation. Someone telephoned Joan's husband and anonymously suggested that a doctor be consulted. It was rather unpleasant to have to make this suggestion but surely Joan's condition was even more unpleasant as it became worse.

Faulty Diet Caused Emotional Upset. A set of tests were made and it was found that Joan had a faulty diet which upset her hormonal balance and triggered off fitful tempers. In addition, she was keeping late hours, disregarding the other natural laws of proper rest, healthful exercise, natural foods, fresh enzyme-rich fruits and vegetables. A special program was developed for Joan to help normalize her hormonal system and also ward off what were unpleasantly considered "senility" symptoms.

Enzyme-Vitamin Nourished Brain. Joan W. was told to begin each meal with a large plate of fresh, raw fruits. The benefit here is that raw fruits are dynamite sources of precious brain-feeding Vitamin C. An enzyme extracts this vital Vitamin C from the fresh, raw fruits and together with oxygen, sends it to nourish the entire body, especially the cells of the brain. The adrenal glands, responsible for nourishing the nerve-brain system, need Vitamin C as found in raw fruits. A youthful brain has a high content of this precious vitamin. Joan W. began her anti-senility program with the enzyme-vitamin power of brain-nourishing fresh fruits.

Protein Feeds and Self-Generates Brain Power. Daily, Joan W. would eat a concentrated protein food. This could be a fat-trimmed piece of meat, fresh water fish, a soft-boiled egg, natural and non-processed cheese, even nuts. Protein is transformed into amino acids by enzymes (found in fresh raw foods) and then sent to nourish the delicate tissues and cells of the brain and body, as well. Protein may well be considered brain food.

The B-Complex Vitamins Create Mental Stability. The B-Complex group of vitamins serve to create mental stability by working together with enzymes to create the process of oxidation in the body and, notably, the brain. That is, the B-complex vitamins assist in carbohydrate oxidation so nerve tissues can remain nourished and are able to "breathe." The nervous-brain system is interlocked and requires an abundant source of this family group of vitamins. Joan W. would take food supplements rich in Vitamin B-Complex to help build up her supply. Or—she could use Brewer's yeast (available at most health stores and special food shops) as well as wheat germ for a power-packed supply of the nerve-brain Vitamin B-complex. Daily, she would use these food supplements.

The Vitamin to Feed the Nervous System. Because Joan W. was fidgety, easily upset and highstrung, she was told to eat foods rich in a nerve-strengthening vitamin. The valuable Vitamin A is especially good for the nervous system and the brain; it works to feed the epithelial cells that line and cover the network of nerves in the body. Vitamin A also works with the functioning of the hormonal-nervous system in this delicate network. Without it, this network may become degenerated and symptoms of senility may appear. Joan W. ate Vitamin A-containing foods such as fresh raw carrots, fresh calf liver, cod liver oil (a powerhouse of Vitamin A), dandelion greens, turnip greens, fresh spinach. One unusually good benefit is that the B-complex vitamins help the liver to manufacture hormones which certainly influence the brain-nervous system more than other organs. Joan W. was thus able to feed her nervous system the natural way.

BRAIN POWER BECOMES NOURISHED AND INVIGORATED. It took two months of proper adherence to proper diet and healthful natural laws before Joan W. became happy and emotionally stable again. Now she was more youthful and alert than ever before.

But like many other folks who regain health, Joan W. became overconfident. She slid back to her faulty foods, kept late hours, ate sweets in overabundance and generally disregarded the natural laws for abundantly healthful living. Now she became more distressed and nervous than before. When last heard of, she had to go to a rest home and recovery may be prolonged, if it comes at all. Perhaps she will learn the one inviolate law of Nature—*What you eat today—thinks tomorrow*!

Morning Brain Boost Beverage

George T. is one of those types who feel sluggish in the morning. He has a difficult time getting out of bed, and finds it even more difficult to get to work on time. To add to George's distress, it takes an hour before he is able to get started at his draftsman's table in the engineering office where he works. George T. has to rely upon caffein-containing coffee and sweetened pastries for his so-called energy boost. True, he gets a boost but the sugar metabolism and caffeine spurt are so rapidly metabolized that after a high energy spurt, he drops down again to his lassitude and lethargy. His co-workers kept ribbing him about his late hours and hangover.

How All-Natural Beverage Boosted Brain Power. When George T. found himself falling behind schedule, and when threatened with a possible dismissal from his job, he decided to get himself examined. His living habits and eating habits were discussed and a program was outlined. Since his basic problem was the lethargy of early morning, often called "morning syndrome" or "morning hangover" caused by poor hormonal-brain function, a special all-natural beverage was suggested.

Each morning, *before* breakfast, George T. would drink this beverage. Then he would have a breakfast of a seasonal raw fruit, a soft-boiled egg or whole grain cereal with milk, and a dessert with a cereal coffee or what is known as coffee substitute. He followed the program and was soon bouncing out of bed with an eager desire to work ahead. The rewards were obvious. He was soon promoted. Now, when this particular Morning Brain Boost Beverage is taken, in conjunction with the other natural laws for abundantly healthful living to be followed in the regular health-boosting quest, the brain is given its self-generating power. It is essential to build all of the natural laws into the daily life in order to reap the rewards of abundant and youthful mind power.

MORNING BRAIN BOOST BEVERAGE

½ glass fresh orange juice
½ glass fresh grapefruit juice
2 tablespoons natural honey
Sprinkle of Brewer's Yeast Powder

Stir vigorously and blend together. Drink this all-natural beverage first thing in the morning. Then follow with the all-natural breakfast that worked wonders for George T.

Benefit of Morning Brain Boost Beverage. The secret power lies in the store of Vitamin B-complex, Vitamin C, and also precious minerals such as calcium and phosphorus. In combination, such as with the special beverage taken by George T., the minerals work to facilitate a hormonal flow which, in turn, "sucks up" Vitamin C which then carries oxygen to the "starved" brain. Vitamin B-complex then goes to work, sparked by calcium-phosphorus, to invigorate the lining of the nerve-brain cellular network. In harmony, like a symphony of health, each instrument (vitamin) plays its role in creating a master-piece of vitality and emotional pleasure. Nature works to build natural mental energy with this harmonious family of nutrients. That is, perhaps, the most valuable secret of the Morning Brain Boost Beverage—the unique natural blending of the nutrients to help nourish the nerve-brain-hormone network.

The 9-Step Guide for Melting Mind Fatigue

Corrective foods form the basis for invigorating and nourishing the mind. When followed in conjunction with this 9-step home guide for melting mind fatigue, the entire body enjoys a supercharging of mind-body energy.

The benefit of this 9-step "instant exercise" guide is to unlock clogged and trapped oxygen pockets that turn fetid and into abrasive lactic acid. This latter substance is harsh and volatile and is responsible for gnawing away at the sheath that covers the nervous system. To help nourish the mind, it is beneficial to "milk out" accumulation of lactic acid.

These simple self-energizing home exercises are best done while lying on your back. Practice daily. If you can do them close to noon when mid-afternoon slump is usually felt, it helps offset the accumulation of fatigue-causing lactic acid. It may help banish the mid afternoon slump the natural way.

Follow this 9-step guide daily for overall benefits:

1. Clench both fists. Notice the pull or tenseness on your wrist, around your elbow, and even up in the shoulder. This is extreme muscular tension which has locked in mind-depleting lactic acid.

2. Open your fists. Immediately, the muscles of your hand, forearm, arm and shoulder release their contraction. In so doing, lactic acid is slowly milked out and nourishment is able to travel along the nerve network to the brain.

3. Perform the preceding exercise three times—clench and relax three times.

4. Next, bend the toes and feet downward, and push or stretch downward with the heels. Notice the pull or tenseness in your ankles, feet, hips and thighs, but especially in the calves of the legs. This is accumulated lactic acid or muscular tension that is about to be expelled.

5. Now let go. The muscular tension begins to melt.

6. Do the foot exercise three times. (Repeat Nos. 4 and 5 three times.)

7. The last relaxing exercise benefits the tired feeling in the neck, throat and face. First, close the eyes. Shut them as tightly

as you can. At the same time, press the lips together, and bite hard with the jaws. This contracts the muscles of your eyes, forehead, mouth, jaw and neck. You can easily feel the accumulated tension about the head—and even hear it ringing in your ears.

8. Now let go with your jaw and face. If your head falls to one side, let it. You are learning to release accumulation of tension-causing lactic acid and other toxic wastes. Slowly, you are self-washing your insides so that your brain can receive its stimulating source of fresh oxygen and nutrients.

9. Perform the face and jaw exercises three times (Nos. 7 and 8). You may need to practice several times on this last exercise before you are the master, for of all the body muscles, it is most essential to learn how to relax those in the face and head. When this is done, the nerve-artery network becomes "self-cleansed" and is able to transport fresh and sparkling oxygen and nutrients to the brain. It helps to self-generate a youthful mind.

Special Benefit of 9-Step Guide. By helping to milk out fatigue-causing poisons and eliminating the debris that clogs the routes of brain food, you will have a beneficial sensation of "all-goneness" because of this free-flowing oxygen. You will also feel light and happy and youthfully alert.

How to Test Your Improved Muscle-Brain Liberation. Since taut, constricted muscles indicate possible choked up debris and the inability to transport nutrients and oxygen to the brain, it is essential that you follow these simple home exercises. In order to test the success of the muscle-brain liberation through free-flowing oxygen, have someone lift your arm or leg. Test to see if it is as limp as a dishrag, after you have tensed it three times and "let go" three times. Your head should be easily rolled from side to side. If there is any stiffness or resistance in your arms, legs, or neck, then you still have clogged up debris that is inhibiting the free flow of brain food such as oxygen and the valuable nutrients. You will need to perform the 9-step guide daily, in conjunction with the other natural laws, to help cleanse your insides so that your brain and vital organs can help you regain and retain valuable health.

Herbs Help Release Mental Energy

The ancients were well aware of the youth-building powers of herbs and what they called "medicines from the meadows." Herbalists have long suggested specific "Nature grasses" to help offset conditions of senility and to help cause a free-flowing circulation to nourish the brain and its thinking components.

You can prepare your own Energy Tea in this simple way:

Take ¼ teaspoon of any one of these herbs (available at most herbal pharmacies listed in the classified directory of local telephone books): gentian root, scullcap, colombo, rue, valerian, vervain, peppermint, spearmint.

Steep this ¼ teaspoon in a pot of boiling water. Let cool and drink each day as you would any tea. The magical herb will help improve the circulation and reportedly will unblock debris and permit an internal free-flowing stream of nutrient-carrying oxygen to the brain and other vital organs.

ACTIVATE YOUR SELF-GENERATOR FOR IMPROVED BRAIN POWER. If the body's reserves are carefully nourished and nurtured, they will serve as fuel to cause activation of your own self-generator for brain power. A depletion of vital processes is often reportedly traced to premature senility. This is not an overnight occurrence. Rather, it is a silent, continuous leakage of the vital reserves until, by its sapping influence, it causes a "brain starvation" and senility. By building the various Natural Laws into your life, you can put youth into your body and your mind.

Summary of Main Brain Points

1. To improve oxygenation of the brain, regulate your blood sugar level with the special listing of foods to eat to your brain's content—and foods to eliminate to help wash out your oxygen-carrying nerve-hormonal network.

2. Nutrients that spark brain alertness include Vitamin C, protein, the B-complex family, Vitamin A. All work harmoniously. Note how they helped Joan W. melt symptoms of senility and bounce back to youthful mental power.

3. The Morning Brain Boost Beverage is easy to make, and is a quick source of "instant brain power." It takes minutes to prepare, offers a lifetime of benefits.

4. Melt mind fatigue by milking out accumulation of fatigue-causing lactic acid. The easy 9-step guide is beneficial for self-cleansing and self-energizing.

5. A reported herbal brew, the time-honored Energy Tea, permits self-washing to flush out impurities that may block the route· of oxygen-nutrient traffic attempting to reach and nourish the brain.

6. The corrective food program calls for natural and fresh foods. The inviolate natural law for self-generating brain power is basically this one: WHAT YOU EAT TODAY—THINKS TOMORROW. As a guide in corrective food selection, rember to EAT FOOD THAT IS BORN, NOT MADE!

7

HOW TO EAT TO FEEL YOUNGER

Milton S. suffered wringing stomach cramps after many main meals. His distress was further augmented by a feeling of heart-pounding pressure on his left side. Milton S. was one of those types who have to lie down and rest after mealtime. When he started to doze off just moments after finishing his heavy dessert, his wife became concerned. She knew that Milton S. would refuse to admit that he could no longer eat like a youngster. So she began to improve and correct his eating program.

Milton's wife replaced heavy meat dishes with satisfying vegetable dishes. She would prepare a large bowl of fresh, raw garden vegetables that would stimulate the natural flow of digestive enzymes. Then she would offer a cooked vegetable casserole which would require less digestive power but would offer comparable overall nourishment. Desserts were usually very light, without heavy sauces or creams. Again, this would ease the burden of digestion.

Milton responded with some grumbles about having to give up his heavy meats, but he eventually adjusted. It took a month of corrective food planning (the emphasis was on meatless foods as a basis) before his stomach cramps subsided, his chest pains eased and eating became a joy instead of leading to after-dinner punishment.

But Milton sneaked heavy, greasy, fatty foods during lunchtime so that he succumbed to a severe attack of gastritis in mid-afternoon. Now, requiring hospitalization and expensive medication that created many side effects, he regretted having "fooled" his wife by his secret lunchtime binge of hard-to-digest foods. Milton, it is hoped, learned his lesson the hard way.

Plant Proteins Can Rejuvenate Digestion

A natural law is that what you assimilate is more important than what you eat! For many folks, digestion is a chore. Enzymatic function may become weaker with the approach of the middle years. This is Nature's advance warning to apply several corrective principles for rejuvenation of a sluggish digestive power. Here are several reported helpful discoveries:

Plant Proteins Are Digestive Aids. The benefit of plant or vegetable proteins is in the easier digestive process. A gentler enzyme action is required, thus sparing a "tired stomach" from excessive and overworked function.

Plant Proteins Are Naturally "Clean." Plant proteins are nourished by an all-natural source. Unlike meat proteins, the plant is free from pathogenic bacterial or parasitical contamination.

Plant Proteins Are "Instant" Sources of Digestive Youth. Many who find it difficult to digest and assimilate meat foods, may find that plant proteins provide a feeling of "Instant Digestive Youth" in accordance with the other natural laws of health. The secret of Nature is this: there is little in the protein of the meat that the animal did not derive from the plant. Not being able to synthesize amino acids, the animal merely appropriates these, ready-made, from the plant, in the form of plant proteins. Man can do this as efficiently and as easily as the animals. You can get your proteins directly from the plant for instant and untampered-with assimilation.

Plant Proteins Spare Excess Acid Flow. Grace T. was embarrassed by the hot, burning flow in her stomach, after she would eat a heavy meat meal. She would take the so-called stomach alkalizers, but this upset the natural balance and after the chemicalized effect wore off, she had an even greater "fire" sensation in her stomach. Grace T. might have continued enduring this discomfort had it not been for her daughter-in-law. The younger woman invited her for a week's visit at their country home. Here, Grace T. was given luscious vegetable meals with a modest and less-dominant portion of meat. Grace T. found that vegetables were soothing and comforting. But she noted that excess meat produced this burning sensation. Now Grace T. learned that meats cause a flow of acid; but more pertinent was the fact that meats are acid-forming foods. She was pouring acid upon acid with her pronounced meat program. By balancing and emphasizing fresh raw vegetables, either as a meal, or as a starter on the menu, she caused a natural alkaline flow that helped soothe and comfort her digestion. Grace T. now enjoyed her food because of the good feeling it produced. She also nourished herself with valuable plant proteins. She still enjoys her meat but in lesser quantities. Furthermore, she obeys one basic Natural Law: *begin each meal with a fresh raw vegetable salad to stimulate the flow of digestive enzymes, and to supply the system with a necessary and NATURAL alkalizer.* Grace T. no longer needs drugstore-purchased alkalizing powders. Nature has solved this problem through fresh raw vegetables and plant proteins.

Plant Proteins are Sparkling Fresh and Self-Scrubbing in the Body. Plant foods offer what is known in Nature lore as "clean substances" in contrast to animal or meat foods. It is reported that digestion of meat foods is frequently impaired by substances which the body cannot use and which must be filtered off as waste materials by the liver and kidneys. This internal debris often clogs the delicate tubules of the liver and kidneys and creates a choked-up reaction. This may put a strain on the vital organs. There is also the problem of putrefaction and toxic accumulation. Plant foods are fresh, self-cleansing and contain enzymes that will exert a feeling of "self-scrubbing" to the organs of the system. Naturally alkaline, they soothe and smooth the digestive organism, in contrast to naturally acid meat products which may offer debris-laden burning and discomfort. Plant proteins make eating a gustatory pleasure instead of stomach burning caused by meat-acid proteins.

The European Waerland System for Super-Health

In Europe, and principally in Sweden and Switzerland, there is a movement which teaches new and all-natural methods to regain and maintain super-health. It has come to be known as Waerlandism. It is named after the founder of this all-natural program, Are Waerland.

The Founder of the Waerland System. Dr. Waerland was a Swedish biologist, who fell ill to the ravages of poor health customs. In his early years, Dr. Waerland discarded the natural laws and ate, drank and lived carelessly. When he reached his early middle years, he developed one illness after another. His liver, kidney and heart became infected. He blood pressure soared. He was unable to continue his studies or teaching and lecturing at universities in Sweden, Denmark, Finland and elsewhere in Europe. Now, he became very sick. When told that he had only a short time to live, Dr. Waerland set out to correct his faulty living habits.

Nature Helped Ease Lifelong Ailments. It was Dr. Waerland's discovery that the entire body must be healed, rather than just treating the part. He knew from his own experiences that in his youth, he had received constant and harsh medication to treat the "parts" such as chronic inflammation of the throat, recurring headaches which were almost like migraine, irritation of the stomach accompanied by inflammation. He also suffered from stubborn constipation. Doctors treated these "parts" with medication, yet the "whole" was ignored. Now, when he developed a painful case of colitis and appendicitis, he started on his own quest for the natural laws of abundantly healthful living. He turned to Nature and prepared this three-step program for himself and, later on, for his many thousands of followers:

1. Foods should be consumed in their natural state. The more natural the food, the greater the successful restoration and retention of super-health.

2. A lacto-vegetarian food program helps invigorate and supercharge the ailing organism with renewed health.

3. Raw foods are living foods and therefore are able to

provide living nutrients to the body. Fresh raw fruits and vegetables and raw grains—untampered with by processing—have the healing power to restore the *entire* body, which is the goal of super-health.

Nature Creates Miracle Cure for Dr. Waerland. By following the basic natural laws with the three-step plan above, Dr. Waerland was able to create self-cure. This drugless healing was brought about by giving the body its natural flow of power through natural food and corrective living habits. Where drugs and medications worsened Dr. Waerland's condition, Nature self-cleansed, healed and rejuvenated. Now, he was completely cured by Nature. He continued in his research and discoveries well into the eighth decade of his life. He might have continued well over the hundred mark except that he had self-experimented with unnaturally hot baths. Daily, Dr. Waerland would soak himself for an hour in excessively hot tubs in order to perspire profusely. In so doing, he made excessive demands on his heart and he succumbed in the prime of health. He left behind a legacy of health treasure which we shall now explore.

The Benefit of Raw Food for Internal Cleanliness

How Raw Foods Cleanse Intestine. Dr. Waerland discovered from scientific demonstrations that raw foods create a self-cleansing intestinal benefit. He explained to the many hundreds of thousands before whom he lectured, that when a man ingests cooked foods, warnings are immediately given to the intestinal canal so that its walls become occupied by leucocytes (white blood cells). This creates an imbalance with red blood cells. The influx of leucocytes to the intestinal walls to help defend the organism against cooked foods causes a clogging of the walls. Consequently, there is an internal clutter that may infiltrate and adversely irritate other adjoining organisms, not to mention the bloodstream. Dr. Waerland suggested that the diet be composed basically of raw vegetables. The familiar suggestion again appears an an inviolable law of Nature: EAT FOOD THAT IS BORN—NOT MADE. Further, cook *only* those foods which *must* be cooked and cannot be eaten raw.

Why Dr. Waerland Urged Drinking of Sour Milk. The doctor explained that man belongs to the mammals and that milk, even though it comes from animals, should be consumed. But he suggested "sour milk," which we today know as yogurt, for these benefits:

Yogurt Creates Self-Detoxification. Dr. Waerland found that sour milk or yogurt is beneficial because it improves assimilation and self-cleanses the colon of putrefactive bacteria; simultaneously, it increases the number of essential bacteria that will help the colon to open the cellulose and digest its contents.

Yogurt Hastens Production of Body's Self-Defenses. The natural milk sugar of yogurt passes into the colon where it hastens production of lactic acid which is needed as the body's self-defense. This intestinal lactic acid then serves to neutralize the harsh acidific effects of putrefactive wastes. It is a form of self-defense against accumulated toxic wastes.

How Milk Improved Vegetable Healing Power

Dr. Waerland tells of a young woman, Inge B., who may have been in her twenties but looked like a woman in her sixties. She came to him for help when she was already showing signs of declining health. Her face was wrinkled, her hair was stringy, she was stoop-shouldered and her eyes were glassy and vague, Inge B. was nervous, easily irritated and on the verge of a collapse. Dr. Waerland immediately put her on this program:

1. All foods should be eaten fresh and raw.
2. Meats, fish, eggs, in moderation.
3. Fresh fruit and vegetable juices throughout the day.
4. All artificial foods were eliminated. This included pastries, rich desserts, artificial sauces, gravies, sweets, etc.

Dr. Waerland again emphasized for Inge B., as he had for thousands of others who recovered health through natural means, that "the more the foods are left in their original state, the more valuable they are for maintaining sound health."

Inge B. Has Partial Health Restoration. In four weeks, Inge B. began to feel better. Her skin looked younger, her hair was thicker, her posture was normal and she had a youthful look about her. But she still felt constant fatigue, had nervous outbreaks and was generally depressed. Dr. Waerland then suggested a unique but highly effective way to use milk to stimulate and improve the nutritive power of vegetables.

How a Vegetable Can Be "Cooked" by Milk

Dr. Waerland was not stubbornly opposed to the cooking of fruit or vegetables, but explained that they lose much of their value when fire-treated. He suggested that vegetables be "cooked" by milk. He put Inge B. on this special program.

How to "Milk" Cook Vegetables: Replace the cooking of vegetables with fresh milk. That is, any vegetable which should be cooked can be prepared by placing it for a certain time, from 15 minutes to several hours, in milk.

Benefit of "Milk" Cooking Vegetables:: The benefit is that no vitamins or other essential nutrients are lost as in the case of cooking by fire and in a pot of water. Dr. Waerland suggested that the milk should also be used as a beverage. The time that the vegetable should "cook" or soak in milk depends upon taste and class of vegetable. For example, horseradish needs several hours. Cauliflower needs from 15 to 30 minutes. Dr. Waerland recommended using sour milk or yogurt for this natural cookless cooking. Others have found that fresh milk can be just as suitable. It is a matter of taste. Needless to say, there is *no* heating of the milk. Just soaking at room temperature!

Inge B. Discovers Renewed Youth. When Inge B. followed this all-natural program, she responded with a miraculous youth renewal, It took five months but Inge B. became younger until she was lovely enough to be taken for an adolescent. Nature had rewarded her with the blessing of youth and abundantly healthful living. Dr. Waerland was happy to be of help.

The Basic Waerland Food-for-Health Program

Dr. Waerland suggested the following five-step food-for-health program:

1. A daily supply of fresh raw fruits and vegetables.

2. Whole grain bread products.

3. Modest cooked fruits and vegetables, where taste and habit call for this preparation. Either standard fire-water cookery or the preceding "milk cooking" process.

4. Fresh raw fruit and vegetable juices daily.

5. The health-building all-Natural foods of Kruska, Molino, Excelsior. (Dr. Waerland's recipes follow in this same chapter.)

FOODS EXCLUDED FROM WAERLAND PROGRAM. Dr. Waerland's program succeeded when his patients and followers could comfortably obey the dictum of a meatless fare. But for those who found it difficult, modest portions of meat, eggs, fish could be consumed in order to provide overall personal satisfaction, But the following items had to be eliminated in order for the body to be able to marshal its self-healing forces:

Items to Be Excluded: common salt, white sugar, white flour and all its products, tobacco, alcohol, coffee, cocoa, tea.

The Three "Waerland Wonder Foods"

The basic foundation for health restoration called for nourishing the body with three fundamental "Waerland Wonder Foods," as his patients and followers called them. These should be made from all-natural and chemical-free items.

KRUSKA. Mix equal portions of whole grain of wheat, rye, barley, oats and millet. Grind thick. To this, add natural raw wheat bran in a proportion of one-half of the amount of the other mixture. Boil in water for 5 to 10 minutes in an open saucepan without lid. Just enough water should be used so that after boiling, the Kruska is creamy. Now place in a covered kettle and keep in a warm room temperature. Let remain for two hours until it becomes expanded. The longer it remains, the more healthful it becomes through a natural enzymatic action.

How To Eat Kruska: Eat with fresh milk, or fruit slices, according to taste.

Benefit of Kruska: Helps regulate and normalize digestive system. The absence of cellulose and plant fibre means constipation, the bran of Kruska absorbs moisture and thus keeps the liquid in the bowels. Bran and the other grains in Kruska stimulate the peristalsis and increase the waves of rhythmic contractions and expansions so necessary for "internal vitality."

Rich Mineral Supply: Kruska is a treasure of such blood and nerve building minerals as iron, iodine, potassium, phosphorus. It is reported that Kruska contains 12 times more combinations with phosphorus than white or refined sulphuric-acid bleached flour.

Rich Vitamin Supply: Appreciable amounts of Vitamin A, B-complex and Vitamin E in Kruska help nourish and enrich the bloodstream and billions of body tissues and cells.

Kruska Provides Strength and Energy: Dr. Waerland found that the rich nutrient treasure in Kruska helped provide strength and energy to the laborers and workers in the field, especially those in the rugged mountains and forests of northern Sweden. He found that when these hard laborers were given daily Kruska portions, they showed more strength than on meat!

MOLINO. The second "Waerland Wonder Food," Molino, is made as follows: Prepare a mixture of 2 spoonfuls of linseed, 2 of wheatbran, 1 spoonful of crushed wheat or unbleached flour of Graham, 3 shredded figs and a handful of raisins. Boil in 1/3 pint of water for 5 minutes. When lukewarm, remove and eat with milk or stewed fruit. (NOTE: The wheat and raisins should be natural and unbleached and free from chemical preservatives.)

Benefit of Molino: Dr. Waerland found that the rich, natural carbohydrate supply nourished the nervous system and was gently soothing to the digestive apparatus, thus becoming a natural source of energy.

Soothes a Nervous Colon: Dr. Waerland reported treating Lars F., a young man who suffered from an embarrassing condition of colitis (irregular bowel habits). The constant drain of harsh laxative salts and cathartics depleted his health to the extent that Lars was easily fatigued, developed unsightly skin blemishes, had unpleasant mouth and body odor, and was furthermore developing what Dr. Waerland considered "premature arthritic tendencies." He placed himself under Dr. Waerland's care, utilized the natural programs with modest amounts of meat, eggs and fish. But the mainstay was to use Molino thrice daily. He was also told to eliminate and give up all artificial stimulants and laxatives. He remained on this health restoration program for seven weeks.

Lars was then examined and reportedly had a contented colon! Not only was he regular, but he had actually become healthfully young. His skin glowed, his energy was limitless, his bones and joints moved with the resilient flexibility of a youngster. Lars was pronounced cured. Dr. Waerland reports that it was Molino that established normal regularity and thereby promoted a natural assimilation of nutrients through the use of natural foods. Lars had actually restored Nature to his body and mind. Had he disregarded the natural laws for abundantly healthful living, he would have been an old man at 30! One can only hopefully imagine what this Waerland System can do for oldsters in helping to turn back the Aging Clock.

EXCELSIOR. This third Waerland Wonder Food is one that was used to normalize the acid-alkaline system, the foundation for youthful health. Here is how Dr. Waerland recommended making Excelsior:

Place potatoes in their jackets (well-washed and without sprouts, without chemical residue or sprays), celery and carrots in a kettle, with the potatoes forming at least half the total amount. Add enough water to cover. Boil for 30 minutes without including the time taken to bring to a boil. In other words, the Excelsior should boil—bubbly boil— for 30 minutes.

Now pour off the liquid. *Drink this from ½ to 1 pint of liquid, lukewarm, first thing in the morning. Dr. Waerland* recommended that Excelsior be prepared the night before and then sipped after being reheated to lukewarm, the next morning. The rest of the Excelsior is to be taken throughout the day.

Unique Benefit of Excelsior: The enviable digestive power of a youngster is in his acid-alkaline normalcy. Dr. Waerland recognized this and suggested that Excelsior be taken by grownups because of its high alkaline-producing ingredients.

Unpeeled potatoes, being alkaline, are the basis of Excelsior.

The other ingredients offer taste satisfaction, but the potato forms the alkaline source that restores youth to the digestive system!

Your Alkaline Cocktail

Dr. Are Waerland found that there were two ordinary vegetables which combine in a tasty beverage and create a soothing. coating and self-satisfying reaction upon the digestive apparatus. Here is how to make it:

Mix equal portions of freshly squeezed cabbage juice with cucumber juice. A vegetable juice extractor is the quickest method to use. Stir vigorously. Drink ½ pint to help ease any burning sensation.

Dr. Waerland reported that the benefit of this all-natural Alkaline Cocktail was in the high mineral and potassium content of the raw vegetables, which served to soothe and relax the digestive system and also to ease the flow of hot acid rains that pelt the stomach's insides with a burning stab. The Alkaline Cocktail was a boon to the many thousands who were healed by the Waerland System.

How Mother's Milk-Substitute Prolonged Life

You may be familiar with the true life story of the oil millionaire who lived to be well up in his 90's. American doctors had heard of the Waerland System and recognized the youth-properties of mother's milk. But they preferred actual mother's milk. These American doctors were hired by this oil millionaire to keep him alive. While natural nutrition was part of their program, mother's milk in several variations was the real secret for keeping this oil millionaire not only alive but youthfully vital even in his ninth decade.

Basing their treatment on the Waerland system, these doctors would use (so it is claimed) actual donated mother's milk for this elderly oil millionaire. But they also used the Waerland–prepared substitute for mother's milk which reportedly has all the nutritive youth-power of real mother's milk. Here is how

Dr. Waerland suggested making an all-natural substitute for mother's milk:

Boil grated potato, a grated carrot, some grated celery and a little parsley, together with common dill (herb) in a pint of water for 4 minutes. Strain off the liquid. Mix this liquid with the desired amount of cow's milk which, by the way, should be raw and certified milk. (Pasteurized or homogenized milk is unnatural for this program.) For sweetening, sugar of milk may be added. Dr. Waerland suggested that this "mother's milk" be taken as the *first* and *last* meals of the day. When taken as such it provides, according to Dr. Waerland, the identical health-producing and longevity-producing properties of protective mother's milk.

The oil millionaire reportedly followed this program, together with other natural laws based upon those of Dr. Waerland and described in this book, and was rewarded by living healthfully, happily and youthfully—until his mid 90's.

The Waerland Program for Abundant Health

Generally speaking, Dr. Waerland called for all-natural methods as described throughout this volume. But here are several other pertinent health-beneficial suggestions that were offered by Dr. Waerland:

1. *Rest after the meals to improve assimilation.* Dr. Waerland recommends a rest after a meal. During the early digestive process, the liver delivers to the blood an enzyme which produces a tired feeling. Nature intends for man to rest after meals. The burden that digestion lays on the body is already heavy. To facilitate nutrient-assimilation, it is suggested not to add an "external work" to an already existing "internal work." All animals rest after a meal. They do it by instinct. Dr. Waerland suggested man do it by common sense.

2. *Warmth improves youthful digestive function.* Your body requires warmth for effective digestion-assimilation. For youthful digestion, the blood travels to the stomach and other organs, hence there is a slight chilling effect elsewhere. Many feel rather chilly after digestion is under way. So keep yourself

warm to help improve digestive power.

3. *Eliminate drinking with meals to supercharge digestive function.* Dr. Waerland found that drinking *with* meals can lead to serious digestive malfunctioning. Water or liquids will dilute the enzymes and render them weak.

4. *Liquids should be comfortably warm or cold.* Dr. Waerland found that extremes of heat and cold interfered with the secretion of the digestive juices. Hot drinks weaken and enervate the stomach; they further destroy the tone of the stomach tissues and weaken its power to act and assimilate food nutrients. The prolonged weakening of its tissues in this way often leads to prolapsed (dropped) stomach. Cold drinks stop or inhibit the action of the enzymes which must wait until the temperature of the stomach has been raised to normal before they can resume their digestive action. To shock and chill the stomach is like putting an ice pack on your insides. Dr. Waerland suggests comfortably warm or cold liquids to soothe the digestion.

5. *Drink liquids at least two hours after mealtime.* Dr. Waerland found that water leaves the stomach within about ten minutes after being swallowed. It carries the diluted and weakened juices along with it, thereby interfering with digestion. Dr. Waerland had this suggestion: water or any liquid, taken two hours after a meal, enters the stomach at a time when much digestion is over and the system is ready for liquids. It is always wisest to wait until you feel comfortably digested; a rule of thumb by Dr. Waerland:

> Fruit meals—drink liquids 30 minutes after finishing.
>
> Starch meals—drink liquids two hours after finishing.
>
> Protein meals—drink liquids four hours or more after finishing.

6. *Chew your foods for healthful assimilation.* Dr. Waerland urged proper chewing so that food would be made comfortable for assimilation. He recalls one patient, Helga E., a housemaid, who was always on the go. Helga E. bolted her food, developed chronic colitis, painful headaches and arthritic symptoms. She came to Dr. Waerland on the urging of her employer who valued her as a housemaid. Helga E. followed the programs of the

Waerland system and especially was told to chew her foods properly.

Helga E. experienced a revitalization. Her internal disorders were eased. Her headaches vanished. Her distorted and painful joints were now free flowing and supple.

The benefit here is that when starches and sugars are bolted, fermentation follows. This is because the food is not insalivated and there is no provision in the stomach for digestion of these foods. Not only would Helga bolt down such foods, but she would also wash them down with water. Result? They began to ferment and give rise to toxic acids which made life miserable for her. Chewing and careful eating and abstention from liquids with meals restored Helga to the royal road of health.

But habits die hard. She soon returned to her nervous eating, ate processed foods, had no time to chew raw vegetables. By eliminating Nature, she invited illness. Result? She reappeared in Dr. Waerland's office, a bent over "old" lady, on canes, with an advanced case of arthritis. She was so wracked with pain that her gnarled fingers could scarcely hold the canes. Even sitting down caused a spasm, a cry of pain and a flood of tears.

Now Helga E. implored Dr. Waerland to help her. The doctor sighed as he said that the ravages of neglected illness were so advanced, the best he could offer was partial relief. Had Helga adhered to Nature, her health would have blossomed; instead, it withered and she was like a dying invalid—at the age of just 37.

WAERLAND SYSTEM SAVED THOUSANDS. Under his guidance, Dr. Are Waerland saved the lives of many thousands. By building his program into their daily living, they were able to halt the Aging Clock. But most essential, they gave Nature the raw materials with which to rebuild and regain health. The Waerland System is still being used by followers and healers throughout Scandinavia, Austria, Switzerland and many more countries. Dr. Waerland had visions of a new human race; its people would be rich in health, strength, intelligence. He called it "The Way to a New Humanity." The thousands who reversed aging can well bless the man who symbolized Nature.

Highlights of Chapter 7

1. Plant proteins rejuvenate digestion and help ease stomach cramps. Low in acid and high in alkaline-forming nutrients, plant proteins can be deliciously soothing.

2. The Are Waerland System for Super Health eases lifelong ailments such as arthritis, headaches, colitis, irregularity, skin problems, toxemia, premature aging. The Waerland System is described herein, with case histories and step-by-step programs.

3. The Waerland System calls for "cooking" vegetables in milk for super-health benefits (Lacto-vegetarian system).

4. The five-step Basic Waerland Food-for-Health Program reportedly revitalized and rejuvenated countless thousands of Europeans.

5. Three "Waerland Wonder Foods" are Kruska, Molino and Excelsior, made with simple ingredients. These foods reportedly rejuvenate those who were given up in the prime of life.

6. An Alkaline Cocktail eases problems of acidosis and improves assimilation of nutrients to build health.

7. Dr. Waerland's substitute for Mother's Milk reportedly helped an oil millionaire live well up into his 90's.

8. Fit the Waerland System into your program for abundantly healthful living. It is easy, inexpensive, rewarding!

8

FIVE "MIRACLE" HEALTH-BUILDING NATURAL FOODS FOR BODY AND MIND

Nature created food for healing and for long life. In Nature's garden of health there are many soil-born and sun-nourished foods that are brimming with health-giving benefits. Of this bountiful treasure, let us select five that have reportedly been able to build and rebuild health of mind and body. These five Miracle Health-Building Foods are available at almost any corner market for a modest price. Surely it is wiser and more healthful to look to the corner market for your natural healing, rather than to the corner drug store! Let us now see how five delicious Miracle Health-Building Foods can benefit your mind and body.

Avocado—The Artery Washing Fruit

Adele T. loved her fat but feared the increase of cholesterol. Her doctor cautioned that certain fats (butter, among them) could cause increased cholesterol that could lead to hardening of the arteries. But Adele just had to have satisfaction of her "fat taste buds." She disregarded her doctor's suggestions and continued eating animal fat foods, "marbled" steaks streaked with fat, heavy cream.

Adele developed a serious condition of arteriosclerosis (hardening of the blood vessels) and slowed blood circulation. When a blood test showed an abnormally high cholesterol level (a heavy waxy fat that gathers in crystals along the walls of the gall bladder and vital body arteries), and there was a threat of a heart attack as well as gall bladder distress, she decided to heed her doctor's advice. Now she went on a low-animal fat program and also enjoyed her fat—the avocado way. She soon experienced a reduced cholesterol level, her gall bladder was sparkling clean, her heart was healthful. The avocado had actually "washed" her arteries. In combination with a low-animal fat program, she had been saved from the crippling ravages of a coronary attack, not to mention arteriosclerosis and gall bladder distress. Nature had created this seeming health miracle of artery-washing.

Why the Avocado is a Miracle Healer

What is the avocado? This is a lovely green fruit that grows on large leafy trees in California and Florida. Also known as avocado pear or alligator pear, it is composed primarily of water and unsaturated fat or oily substance which makes it smooth as butter, delicate in texture and flavor. The bland green "fruit meat" of the avocado has a smooth, creamy, rich texture. It lacks the salty tang of table butter, and so is valuable for the salt-free diet.

Natural way to control your appetite. The avocado is ideal for weight-reducing; as the only fruit with a 17 percent concentration of fat, the avocado cuts appetite, slows digestion, helpfully gives a satisfied feeling of having eaten well and plentifully. The avocado contains only 165 calories per 100 grams as compared with butter which contains 733. Green butter (avocado spread) on whole grain bread is more than a tasty treat; it is ideal for the weight loser for it suppresses appetite. One compulsive eater, Gene R., was getting dizzy from prescribed diet, appetite depressing pills. He had narcotic effects under the chemical appetite suppressants. Gene R. gave up his diet pills, then started to eat whole grain bread with a thick spread of avocado "meat." He found that it could control and even eliminate his compulsive eating. This drugless way eased his runaway appetite, helped melt pounds and slim him down.

To remain slim and avoid eating temptations, Gene R. still eats avocados regularly.

Avocado oil washes the vascular-artery system. The avocado has a rare oil seldom found in other fruits. This oil is in a form that is highly digestible. It also contains valuable fatty acids that help wash the vascular-artery network. For the person prone to arteriosclerosis (hardening of the arteries), high blood cholesterol or impaired circulation, avocados are a boon. They help lower the fat content of the blood and excess deposit formation of cholesterol. The avocado can stem the tide of blood vessel disease through its self-washing oil.

Avocados are hearty for heart-saving. This green fruit contains little or virtually no salt, so heart-conscious folks will welcome it as a safe food. Because the avocado is so low in salt, it is ideal to help reduce weight, ease strain on the heart and provide a healthful condition. Those on a low-sodium (salt) health restoration plan would do well to enjoy the benefits of this low-sodium natural fruit.

The fruit that helps build recovery from diabetes. The diabetic should know that the avocado is a fruit, yet it contains very little sugar and almost no starch. It has about 5 percent carbohydrate as compared with other sugar-containing fruits which have up to 20 percent. Because diabetics are likely to run high cholesterol levels, they benefit from the anti-cholesterol or fat-washing effect of avocados.

The beauty benefits of Nature's fruit. Noted cosmetologists and dermatologists have found avocado oil ideal for face, hand and skin creams because of its light texture, which keeps the skin from drying and also helps heal blemishes, those aging marks that distress the adult as well as the youngster. Just spread avocado oil onto the skin blemishes and let Nature soak in the precious oils that help create inner healing as well.

The gourmet food for ulcer people. Doctors reportedly herald the avocado as a gourmet food for the ulcer person; its oils are soothing to an angry stomach and a duodenal ulcer. It is soft, easily digested. Its natural oily content is healing to the inflamed and tender tissues of the stomach lining. Furthermore, the avocado oil cuts down gastric-acid secretions, slows motility and eases the grinding motions of the stomach. To help heal ulcer conditions, discuss this gourmet food with your doctor.

Speeds up healing processes. The bland avocado oil is easily digested by the ailing; even a surgical patient reportedly usually tolerates the avocado without gas or digestive upset. It is an effective and reportedly safe food for a convalescent who has had a gall bladder removal. It can be eaten in place of other fatty foods. To restore strength and vitality, the avocado is versatile and has a satisfying taste.

Live longer on the avocado. A physician reports, "I well recall my grandmother, a rugged little lady who ate an avocado nearly every day and reached the ripe old age of 90. We attributed her longevity and her elastic arteries to the avocado and other nutritious foods. Interestingly enough, though she had no gall bladder, she had no difficulty digesting avocados, whereas some other fatty and fried foods gave her distress." This cholesterol-free fruit may well be Nature's secret for long life.

FEAST ON NATURE'S MIRACLE FRUIT. The juicy goodness of the avocado makes it a feast of health. You may eat the avocado "as is" or chop and dice and use it in a salad. It is best to eat it in a natural state to benefit from the abundance of vitamins, minerals and self-washing oils. Look to Nature for foods that can help you regain and retain abundantly healthful living.

Banana—The Magic Health Builder

Gerald P. loved food—but his stomach did not! Here was a maritime engineer who feared the development of stomach ulcers. Everything he ate was a digestive nightmare. He would experience hot burning stabs in his stomach just an hour or two after an average meal. Furthermore, Gerald P. found himself awakening in the middle of the night with such churning stomach sensations that he felt like screaming from pain. He was so doused with chemical patent medicines, he felt there was nothing to do but suffer.

A ship's electrician suggested fruit but Gerald P. felt even greater gastric distress from most fruits. But when he tried the banana, he experienced a welcome feeling of stomach contentment. Now he began to eat bananas daily.

Benefit of the banana on the digestive system: The ability of the banana to neutralize or buffer free hydrochloric acid, together with the fruit's bland consistency, soft texture and low residue, makes it soothing for ulcerous or stomach conditions. In laboratory tests with a dilute solution of free hydrochloric acid and banana pulp, in just 15 minutes an average of about one-half of the acid disappeared; in two hours, about two-thirds of it was gone. The banana has this buffering action that is happily soothing to the stomach-troubled person.

Gerald P. felt "cured" and gave up his banana with the result that his distress returned with such a hot shower of rains that he now required hospitalization. Had he adhered to Nature and not grown overly and foolishly self-confident, he could very well have been rewarded with a healthy stomach. The banana is well regarded as Nature's miracle fruit.

What is the banana? It is a golden yellow fruit, packaged by Nature in individual germproof containers. No worry about sprays, bacteria or dust reaching the fruit. The banana is easy to peel, the "package" is disposable but don't throw it on the floor, where someone may slip on the peel! It's the easiest fruit in the world to eat. No knife. No napkin. No utensils. Simply peel and enjoy it.

A welcome food for the allergic. Because the banana causes few allergic reactions, it is medically used in diets for the allergic person—whether he is suffering from a skin rash, asthmatic or respiratory-pulmonary conditions or digestive disorders.

Slim down with the banana. This fruit has considerable natural bulk to satisfy the craving for food, yet it has a mere 88 calories per average size banana. The quick energy of the banana's natural fruit sugar puts a quick stop to hunger pangs. One physician who helped reduce weight in patients had this to say, "A diet having as its basis *bananas and milk* is proposed for the treatment of overweight, on the grounds of simplicity, low cost, ready availability, palatability, high satiety value, low salt content and demonstrated effectiveness in securing the desired aim. "

Good news for sodium-restricted persons. Bananas are very low in sodium and are often prescribed for those with problems of the heart, kidney or blood pressure. The less sodium eaten, the less fluid accumulates in the tissues so the low-sodium banana can be good news for health and taste.

The banana causes natural self-washing. The banana has a high amount of potassium, a mineral that helps wash the vital organs such as the kidneys in a beneficial manner.

A natural source of youthful energy. The highly digestible sugar content of ripe bananas is quickly converted into body energy; bananas also have an alkaline effect on the body which facilitates carbohydrate metabolism for speedy and natural energy. A secret for the excellent utilization of banana sugars may be the softness of the fruit's fiber, the bulky residues produced by pectins, the alkalizing action of the fruit on the intestinal contents and the slow release of the carbohydrates.

Heart-soothing effect of the banana. Because bananas are free from cholesterol and contain only a trace of unsaturated fatty acid, they are said to be heart-soothing for the person cautious about the heart and coronary arteries.

How the banana rebuilt youthful health. A physician has this to report: "Some years ago I treated a patient who suffered from a serious case of *anorexia nervosa.* She had reached a serious state of depletion and weakness from her self-imposed starvation, refusing all food and regurgitating (throwing up) what was fed to her. She finally accepted a banana, with the result that other food was taken in a more or less normal amount within 48 hours. There was a complete relapse when the banana was withheld, and food was taken normally only with bananas. Gradually (on a banana program), her appetite was normal whether bananas were included in the diet or not." The patient regained her happy, naturally calm youth. All this could be attributed to the Nature-induced benefit of vitamins, minerals and enzymes in the precious banana.

The banana helps spare protein reserves. The carbohydrate of the banana is highly digestible and also protein-sparing. This action is maximally beneficial where protein and carbohydrates are ingested simultaneously.

The banana establishes normal internal regularity. The semi-solid texture of the banana is attributable to the way its natural sugars, moisture and other nutrients are held in a cellular and pectin meshwork. Both the fiber and the pectin exert significant regulative and protective action in the intestinal tract. The carbohydrate fibrous content and pectin add notably to the bulk produced in the gastrointestinal tract and lead to a sensation of repletion or satisfaction. The banana may well be regarded as a natural laxative!

THE FRUIT WITH THE GOLDEN HOPE OF HEALTH. Delightful as a hand-eaten fruit, in salads, with dessert, the bright yellow golden hope of health belongs in your program to establish harmony with Nature. Easy to eat, easy to assimilate, easy to build your health with.

Grain Foods—Foundation of Strength

Just to talk to salesclerk Janice E. was to get involved in an argument. Janice E. was one of those types who had to eat and run to catch the commuter bus in the morning in order to be in the store on time. She ate dehydrated breakfast foods, bleached bread products and so-called convenience dishes. Janice E. endured mid-morning slump, nervous outbursts, flushed face and goose-pimply skin. When her temper finally cost her job, she decided it was time to find out what was wrong. It is always sad that folks wait until their health (and job) is lost before seeking help.

Janice E. was found to be a sad case of nutritional nerves. The devitalized breakfast food and "dead" grain products had actually depleted her supply of precious B-complex and vitamin E as well as nerve-building minerals and protein. Now she was put on a natural, raw food program with emphasis upon whole grains. But Janice E. followed a partial program. Her nerves were healed but she still had heart palpitations and nervous tremors. Her hands shook so that she could hardly hold a pencil when writing an order on her saleswoman's pad. When Janice E. almost lost her second job, she relied upon Nature all the way with abundant whole grains and natural foods and she regained much of her health. It is hoped she still takes advantage of the healing force in Nature's grasses.

What are grain foods? These include barley, corn, oats, rice, wheat. We generally know them in the form of cereals. The word "cereal" is derived from the ancient Roman ceremonies known as the *cerealia,* celebrated in honor of Ceres, the Goddess of Grain. The festivals, celebrated in Spring, were instituted about 500 B.C. to solicit protection for the growing grain crops. Today, with many grains subjected to bleaching, processing and chemical devitalization, we need to invoke Nature for protection against foodless grains! When selecting any grain food, choose a product that is natural and non-processed. This is a grain product that has retained the specific nutrients of the whole, non-processed grain and which contains natural proportions of bran, germ and endosperm. Health stores have natural grain foods.

Nutrition in a grain nutshell. Natural and non-processed grain is rich in valuable vitamins, minerals, protein and energy-producing carbohydrates. Long before we had food supplemental capsules, our predecessors looked to Nature's own supply in the whole grain food.

The body-building and youth-creating protein of grain. The inner, white part (endosperm) of the wheat berry represents about 80 percent of the whole, and consists of energy-producing carbohydrate and protein. Whole grain proteins are considered of good quality. Doctors report that proteins of whole grain foods are vital for body growth, reproduction, skin, bone and blood-building benefits.

Nerve-building vitamins are nourished in whole grains. The nerve and skin lining vitamins of the B-complex group are Nature-nourished in whole grain foods. The B-complex vitamins are found in the aleurone layer of the bran covering which may be removed during processing, hence the value of natural grain. Furthermore, Vitamin E, so valuable for heart regulation and fertility, is found in the embryo or germ of the grain. Again, processing removes this perishable Vitamin E. The natural and non-processed grains will have these valuable vitamins.

Blood-building qualities of grain foods. Whole grain food contains many excellent minerals, but it is an especially rich source of iron which is easily utilized by the body. It is reported that the iron of whole wheat and bran is more effective for hemoglobin formation than that of lean beef, liver or egg yolk.

Natural source of energy. Whole grains contain carbohydrates which are naturally converted into body sugars to provide good energy. Start the day right with a bowl of any natural and non-processed whole grain food. Packaged or processed "breakfast foods" that are enriched are devitalized, chemicalized and artificially flavored and may deplete rather than build health. The emphasis is upon a *natural* whole grain. Inquire at a local health food shop for non-processed grain foods.

Healthful food for "low-fat" dieters. Whole grains provide low-fat content and are devoid of cholesterol. Those on a low-fat program would do well to include whole grains for taste and for health!

Grains energize the metabolism of nutrients. For carbohydrates and sugars to be metabolized and assimilated by the body for the end products of nerve strength, energy and youthful vitality, a supply of the B-complex vitamins are required. These precious vitamins are in abundance in whole grains. When you eat a whole grain food, you are providing your body with eventual natural vitalic energy through the metabolism that is sparked by B-complex vitamins.

GRAINS ARE FOUNDATION OF YOUTHFUL HEALTH. Highly nutritious and natural, non-processed grains can well form the foundation upon which you build youthful health, in accordance with the other natural laws of abundantly healthful living. Grains benefit health by providing fuel to ignite your built-in source of vitality.

Papaya—Magic Melon of Nature's Medicine

Frank T. found himself in a condition of declining health.

His physician said he had a slight condition of diabetes, as well as anemia. His problem was that intake of sugar as well as some of the minerals which build blood could not be properly assimilated. A build-up of sugar and a blood-starvation of iron created a serious decline of general health. To make it worse, Frank T. loved to eat the very foods that were now restricted. His physician suggested drug medication which created so many side effects that he wondered which was worse, the illness or the medicine!

A neighboring nurse suggested that he strike at the core of his problem—namely, that he boost his assimilation process. She urged fresh fruits which Frank tried, with moderate benefits. But it was the papaya fruit that actually turned the trick. Frank T. ate several fresh papayas daily with the benefit that his enzyme-assimilation process was regenerated, and now the precious minerals could be assimilated to enrich his bloodstream. His condition of diabetes was also relieved but he required modest medication as a precaution. He hopes that papaya and other general and natural health secrets will soon eliminate drug taking.

What is the papaya? This Magic Melon of Nature's Medicine is known as a "tree melon" because of its resemblance to a melon. Actually, this fruit grows on a giant herbaceous plant and not on a tree. It is a tropical fruit and flourishes in Florida, the lower Rio Grande Valley section of Texas and in Hawaii, among other Eden-like surroundings.

How the papaya can nourish a youthful skin. This Magic Melon contains more Vitamin C than oranges. But most astonishing is that this Vitamin C content actually increases as the papaya ripens. It is also reported that daily eating of the papaya can create a similar collagen-forming healing in the body's connective cells and tissues for the look and feel of youthfulness. Ordinarily, Vitamin C is not stored in the body, but coming from the papaya, it may develop a foundation to help nourish and put bloom onto a skin that looks and feels young.

A tasty fruit for the allergic. Because the papaya is extremely bland, there are no known allergies from its consumption. It can be used as a baby's first fresh fruit and for adults who may otherwise have allergic tendencies.

How the papaya fruit helps in nutrient assimilation. One Nature-created ingredient is the enzyme known as *papain*. This is a powerful nutrient-digesting enzyme found exclusively in this Magic Melon. It helps the body enzymes release the nutritional potency in foods for energy and health.

How the papaya can rejuvenate aging digestion. Its supply of papain and other enzymes helps in the digestive process when there may be problems of adequate enzyme function, such as in advanced years. Interestingly enough, Columbus reported that natives ate great quantities of meat and fish and topped these off with papaya. Instinctively, natives knew the papaya aided digestion. Truly, it was a Magic Melon to those who knew nothing about stomach problems because of this wondrous fruit of the tropics.

The almost-human factor in the papaya. This is a strange miracle fruit because of its almost-human factor. It has male and female plants. Its fruit, like the human embryo, develops fully in about nine months. It was heralded by explorer Vasco de Gama as the "golden tree of life," and by Ponce de Leon who called it *Vanti,* which means "keep well." Marco Polo reportedly used it as a staple food for his sailors. Even Magellan prized its life-giving benefits. We may well consider the papaya as a Child of Nature!

ENJOY NATURE'S OWN YOUTH MEDICINE. Papaya is a juicy good, luscious melon-shaped fruit that grows in clusters in the tropics. It is brimming with peculiar and magical juices that may be regarded as Nature's "youth medicine." It is ready to eat when the color ranges from full yellow-orange to yellow green and the fruit flesh yields to gentle pressure of the palms. It should be eaten while the flesh is tender but still firm. The smooth flesh has little fibre, and features a tantalizing aroma and flavor that add up to delicious "medicine" from Nature. It is good as fresh fruit by itself, or in a salad. It is especially beneficial as a dessert when food is to be digested and assimilated to build youthful health.

Soybeans—The "Meatless" Meat

Perhaps no single natural food has produced a greater benefit on world nutrition than the soybean. A native of China, it was first introduced to America some 150 years ago. Today we recognize the soybean as being the most "meatless meat" available for those who wish to have the protein and nutrition of meat without its byproducts or acid-ash residues.

The nutrition power packed in a bean. Soybean has iron, calcium and B-complex and contains all known essential amino acids of protein. It is about 40 percent protein, itself. Soybean is the richest food in potassium, a mineral needed to regulate nerve processes and to help maintain a proper water balance in the body. It features 96 percent available iron, a boon to those who need blood-building benefits.

The soybean helps reduce cholesterol. One welcome benefit is that the soybean is 51.5 percent linoleic acid, an essential fatty acid that is helpful in emulsifying blood cholesterol so it does not form unhealthful deposits.

Effective milk substitute. Stephen F., an overworked real estate specialist, found himself nervous, on edge, always biting his nails. He needed more calcium-phosphorous, the minerals that soothe the nerves. But Stephen disliked milk. He might have continued depriving himself of precious nerve building minerals, had he not tried soybean milk. (It is available at most health stores, or powder is available from which you make your own milk.) Stephen F. found that the calcium in soybean milk is comparable to that of cow's milk. Now he had the nutrition of milk but not from an animal source.

How soybeans can create inner-building of health. Since soybeans are the only meatless food that contain *all* essential amino acids, they can be eaten, reportedly, in place of meat. It might be mentioned that meat is otherwise the only other food with all these basic amino acids. Now, what can soybean amino acids do for your health? Here are some rewards for enjoying this meatless meat:

1. Soybean amino acids are building blocks that serve as the materials of growth, repair and rejuvenation within the body.

2. The body tissues and cells use soybean amino acids for the manufacturing of many body enzymes, for producing hormones and other inner products. It is believed that soybean amino acids assist in production of antibodies to build resistance to the ravages of illness.

3. Soybean amino acids make blood proteins. These feature colloidal osmotic pressure which creates strong, rich blood.

4. Soybean amino acids create energy in the form of split-off amines that are stored to be later used as glucose or glycogen for vital energy.

5. Soybean amino acids enter into the formation of strong bone marrow which stores minerals and helps keep the skeleton structure in a free-flowing form, without arthritic tendencies.

FOR OPTIMUM HEALTH, REMEMBER THE PERFECT MEAT SUBSTITUTE. Many have attested to the life-giving benefits of soybeans, with its meat-like taste and nutritional treasure. As a miracle health-building food, the soybean is the staple and often the only food for millions of people in Asia. When the soybean is used as a meat substitute it offers the benefits of the meat nutrients.

Important Points of Chapter 8

1. Nature has created many miracle health foods in a natural state. This chapter reveals the benefits of five special all-natural foods for regaining and retaining youthful health at all ages.

2. The *avocado* reportedly controls appetite, washes the arteries, benefits the heart, creates digestive power and promotes vibrant physical health.

3. The *banana* is a golden treasure of benefits. It is tolerated by the allergic; it offers a tasty way to reduce, is low-sodium, energy-producing, spares protein, buffers the digestive juices to guard against burning of excess acid.

4. *Grain foods* provide natural and quick energy, needed bulk, nerve-strengthening vitamins and minerals and blood-building benefits.

5. The *papaya* is Nature's own youth medicine with its powerful enzyme able to provide overall assimilation of nutrients.

6. The   *soybean* is the known "meatless meat" with all the amino acids of meat. It may well be the foundation food for health.

9

CONTROLLED FASTING: NATURE'S LAW FOR REJUVENATION OF YOUR BODY ORGANS

In the days before drugs or surgery, an ancient health technique was used for the healing of many ailments. Clearly recommended in the scriptures of nearly all denominations, this ancient technique is reportedly so potent that in a matter of days it helps to rejuvenate and restore the health of even the most hopelessly afflicted. It has widely been practiced throughout the ages and has been responsible for thousands of seemingly miraculous recoveries. Even today, it is practiced in many areas of Europe and the East. It is slowly coming into its own in America.

HOW FASTING CAN CREATE A FEELING OF YOUTH. This ancient health technique is fasting. It involves no drugs, no surgery, no hospitalization. Yet it has long been considered one of Nature's most effective means of helping to create a feeling of youth through internal cleansing. Controlled fasting calls for the elimination or reduction of most solids. This enables the organism to self-cleanse and flush out accumulated wastes and corrosive acids that may be the cause of health depletion and premature aging. During a controlled fast, non-essential body accumulations, such as uneliminated waste that is stored, begin to break down (through autolysis), are returned to free circulation and then eliminated from the body. This helps wash out the insides to create a sparkling clean and youthfully rewarding health condition.

How Controlled Fasting Can Rebuild Health

Many physicians have noted that after a brief period of controlled fasting there is a feeling of general well-being. Many a doctor suggests controlled fasting for problems of gout, arthritic over load, heart distress, skin blemishes, nervous disorder, catarrh, sinus or respiratory disturbances, chronic cold catching, allergic tendencies. The purpose here is to enable the body to rid itself of offensive toxemia that may be responsible for such discomforts.

Fasting Will Wash Out the Insides. During a condition such as a cold, the natural way to help restore health is to wash out the insides through controlled fasting. Many physicians recommend elimination of most foods, and the drinking of fresh fruit and vegetable juices. The benefit here is that the liquids help wash out internal toxins and impurities and thereby create cleansed insides and eventual health restoration. If good elimination is established before and during the fast, the juice-drinking program will surely create sparkling, youthfully fresh insides.

Fasting Helps Improve Brain Function. Rosalind R. was an active clubwoman. But her problem was that when she had to give a speech before her fellow members, she found her words fumbling and her thoughts sluggish. Rosalind R. would usually make her noon meal the main one of the day. While she ate nourishing food, she still felt "brain sluggish" after the meal, when she had to either give a speech or participate in a discussion. Rosalind R. experienced heart flutters and occasional dizzy spells when she forced herself to participate while she still felt the effects of the main noon meal. It might be mentioned that her woman's club always met for this noon dinner and meeting combined. One afternoon, the menu featured foods she disliked so she passed up the meal and had a glass of tomato juice. She noticed that she was mentally alert, intelligent, and had a sharp awareness of everything that took place during her round-table discussion after the noon dinner which she had passed up. Now she had a clue to her erratic behavior. She planned to eliminate a main noon meal until *after* a meeting when she could digest her food without mental stress. Now she solved the problem of what she feared was "hardening of the brain arteries." Simple. Effective. All-natural!

How Fasting Can Create Emotional Health. Controlled fasting is beneficial during times when the brain is subjected to emotional requirement. Putting it simply, during and after a meal, a rush of oxygen-bearing blood is sent to the digestive organs for enzymatic assimilation of ingested food. This means that the brain is thus deprived of a goodly share of oxygen and blood and thinking capacities are simultaneously reduced. This explains the reduced mental power experienced after a main meal. The brain will benefit by controlled fasting. If you are doing heavy study, preparing for a speech, or otherwise engaging in heavy concentration, you will do well to fast. Controlled fasting sharpens your mind and makes you alert and sensitive to mental effort. You are able to concentrate and think more easily if your stomach is comfortably empty and not drawing blood from the brain to digest food. Emotionally, controlled fasting can help create a youthful energy.

Fasting Can Relieve Digestive Distress. Normal (and abnormal) eating causes a natural but often overworked responsibility of the stomach, liver, pancreas, intestines. Controlled fasting helps give these and other vital digestive organs a well-needed vacation so that self-cleansing will later provide rejuvenated ability.

Helps to Ease Ulcer Tendency. It is reported that when you drink plenty of fresh water and raw vegetable juices during controlled fasting, there is almost no risk of the development of a stomach malady or peptic ulcer. It is further reported that many cases of colitis and intestinal disorder are greatly benefited by a periodic fast, which gives the intestines a chance to rest.

Good News for Diabetics. Physicians who supervise fasting have found that if you take nothing but water during a controlled fast, use *no* sweet drinks or starches, the pancreas is given a well-deserved rest. This large, long organ or gland is located behind the lower part of the stomach. One prime function of the pancreas is to manufacture enzymes and hormones that serve to metabolize carbohydrates. Failure of the pancreas to function efficiently may lead to inadequate supplies of insulin (a hormone) and a condition of diabetes may follow. By following a controlled fast of elimination of all foods and drink except water, there is an easing of the function of the pancreas. It is allowed to self-rejuvenate through a rest. Furthermore, water drinking will help reduce hunger pangs. When hunger disappears, insulin is not required to utilize the glucose in the bloodstream, (glucose produced by large amounts of starchy and sweet foods), and can be used to metabolize accumulated sugar-forming carbohydrates. Diabetics would do well to consider controlled fasting a means of helping to restore internal cleanliness.

Controlled Fasting Helps Rejuvenate the Skin. Those troubled with such skin disorders as psoriasis, acne or aging blotches, are often advised by their physicians to elinimate sweets and fats from their diet. This helps self-cleanse the body and is a form of controlled fasting. It would be best to eliminate all foods for a while and let the skin pores have a chance to cleanse themselves and then put a youthful rosy tint to the cheeks.

Controlled Fasting Gives a Rest to the Heart. A day or two on fresh raw vegetable juices will help relieve the pressure on the heart and circulation. A controlled fast helps eliminate salt and water from the body, reduce tissue edema, regulate normal breathing. This helps to bring about comfortable sleep and an overall hearty good feeling.

How to Begin Your Fast

Prepare for the fast. Several days before the appointed fast day, prepare by reducing all non-essential foods. Eliminate starchy and sweet foods, heavy desserts, excessive eating. Increase your intake of fresh fruit and vegetable juices as well as lots of fresh raw fruits and vegetables in a succulent salad.

Prepare your system for the controlled fast by the slow elimination of heavy foods.

First day: On the first day of your fast, drink lots of fresh raw vegetable juices. If you must have some solids, select succulent and juicy vegetables to satisfy that chewing urge.

Second day: On the second day of your fast, drink lots of fresh raw fruit juices. Again, if you must have something to chew, select good juicy, raw fuits.

Third day: In the morning, two glasses of any desired juice. At noon, drink another two glasses of juice, and in the evening, another two glasses of any desired juice.

Fourth day: Drink only fresh water.

How and When to End Your Fast

The length of the fast is self-determined. Usually, you know by a feeling of lightness and youthfulness that the self-cleansing has been done. That is Nature's reward for controlled fasting. To break the fast, begin with a day of succulent, chewy, good raw vegetables. The next day, follow with juicy good and fibrous fruits. The third day, begin to eat your main foods which may include milk, eggs, fish, meats, beans, etc. Eat modestly to avoid shocking your relaxed digestive apparatus into sudden function. When you establish normal eating, modesty and reason are the watchwords. Again, eat to nourish and not to stuff. Eat food that is *born* and *not made.* Health restoration becomes compatible with Nature.

HOW TO SATISFY HUNGER URGE DURING FAST. The Bedouins, wandering in the desert, reportedly survive for days on a few dates. They satisfy the hunger urge by munching, chewing and pre-digesting dates. The same applies to raisins which offer excellent energy-producing grape sugar. Take a tip from these desert wanderers and satisfy hunger with dates and/or raisins.

BE OF GOOD CHEER DURING FASTING. Happiness is a natural medicine which stimulates the glands and keeps them at the peak of their youthful efficiency. During your fasting, be happy and content. Avoid controversy. Get plenty of sleep.

Take nightly showers or baths in comfortably tepid water. This helps create an internal and external "spring-cleaning" sensation of youth. Just as spring is the herald of approaching youth, so is your internal "spring-cleaning" a rejuvenation of good things to come.

The Waerland System of Renewed Youth Through Fasting

The Swedish naturist healer, Dr. Are Waerland, was able to help renew and restore a feeling of youth among his thousands of followers throughout Europe, through his own unique Waerland System of Fasting.

RAW VEGETABLE JUICE FASTING. Dr. Waerland found that a controlled fast consisting of raw vegetable juices (and no other foods) was able to supply the body with precious healing mineral alkaline substances and vitamins. He found that the outpouring of mineral alkaline substances in the digestive system was able to scrub and wash out accumulated debris and residue. The program that Dr. Waerland recommended for his followers is outlined here:

1. The fast should be of short duration, perhaps two or three days.

2. The fast permits unlimited amounts of fresh raw juices.

3. Dr. Waerland recommended that only alkaline or neutral liquids be consumed, never any acids. Such alkaline liquids include Excelsior (see Chapter 7 for recipe), raw juices from root vegetables, green leafy vegetable juices. The neutral foods included milk and its derivatives and the strained-off liquids of most cooked vegetables. Note that this is still an all-liquid fasting program, recommended by Dr. Waerland. Furthermore, water is also neutral and may be consumed freely during the fast. This is essential since water acts as the carrier for sloughing off and ridding the body of the accumulated waste matter.

THE WAERLAND SYSTEM FOR ENDING A FAST. Dr. Waerland suggests that the first meals after a fast should be carefully selected; the organs of digestion with the big apparatus of muscles and glands have had a complete rest. Therefore, foods that are easily digested should be considered. Dr. Waerland had these recommendations to his followers:

First Meal: Yogurt or sour milk which should be taken with care, in spoonfuls, holding each portion for a while in the mouth to assure a thorough mixture with mouth enzymes.

Second Meal: Mashed potatoes which can be eaten with yogurt or sour milk. Later, whole grain and non-processed rice cooked in water may be included.

Third Meal: Include more solid foods in modest portions. Dr. Waerland, as a lacto-vegetarian, suggested any easily digested dairy or vegetable food as the third meal.

WAERLAND SUGGESTIONS FOR HEALTH DURING FASTING. The doctor suggested that the person who fasts should not do unusually heavy work or make any unnecessary physical exertions. Neither should he stay too long in bed; the fasting person was advised to get up, walk about, enjoy comfortable physical movement. If there is some tiredness, the person should lie down. Avoid cold. Sleeping should be in a well-ventilated room in order to carry out the gaseous eliminations of the lungs and skin.

Reactions Felt During the Controlled Fast. During the self-cleansing, a natural phenomenon takes place. The body cells feed the digestive juices (the reverse of what usually occurs; namely, the digestive juices feed the cells). The body then begins to extract from the cells and tissues the useless and toxic substances that have accumulated. Now the organs of elimination work with greater intensity. The lungs give off an acrid odor; the skin stresses its elimination and eruptions may appear. The tongue is covered by a malodorous coating. The kidneys produce a stronger urine than ever. But the major reaction is that the digestive apparatus works to eliminate wastes.

The colon (an organ of absorption) now becomes an organ of elimination that throws off toxins through its walls. Toxic masses now arrive from the stomach and small intestine. The liver sends a bile to the intestine that is saturated with toxins and useless substances. Furthermore, excess fat becomes metabolized and its acrid end products are given off. These are some of the reactions noted amongst those who have extreme health decline and prolonged internal sludge accumulation.

Benefit from Successful Controlled Fasting. Slowly, the breath becomes fresh. The tongue is clean. The eyes are clear. The skin is youthful and rosy. The urine is amber in color. These indications announce that Nature has helped the body cleanse itself and improve youthful health.

Dr. Waerland explained that controlled fasting helped the body to scrub out debris through the basic six organs of elimination: the colon, kidneys, skin, lungs, liver and mucous membranes. These six organs are then self-cleansed and self-washed and help the body regain and retain abundantly healthful living. The natural law of fasting has been fulfilled.

A DOCTOR'S REPORT ON FASTING. One noted physician had this to report to a medical journal, "Not long ago I tried a five-day fast (for weight reduction). The most impressive finding was lack of fatigue and freedom from hunger after 48 hours. *I actually felt sharper mentally, and was able to perform heavy surgical operations with skill and mental alertness equal to that which I had when eating.*

"A feeling of euphoria (lightheadedness and happiness) is noted by some people on a fast, and this was my experience. I actually felt peppier and more alert mentally. I slept more soundly than when eating regularly."

AN ALL-NATURAL POTASSIUM BROTH. Because fasting calls for much washing out of wastes, the body may be depleted of a valuable kidney-washing mineral, potassium. It is reported that the person going on a fast should sip a cup of warm vegetable broth in the evening. This helps take the sting out of missing the evening meal, supplies the body with this magic mineral, potassium, and also boosts a feeling of energy and vitality.

FEEL YOUNG THROUGH CONTROLLED FASTING. This ancient drugless health technique is slowly becoming the key to rejuvenation in our modern times. It provides a feeling of well-being, a clearer eye, sharper brain, springier step and greater work efficiency. It helps the flow of youth bloom anew.

It is one of the most ancient and popular laws for abundantly healthful living. It's free!

Summary of Vital Points in This Chapter

1. An ancient drugless health technique is coming into its own in our modern times. Controlled fasting is enjoying a rebirth.

2. Controlled fasting, among other benefits, reportedly washes out the insides, stimulates brain function, creates emotional youth strength, relieves chronic digestive distress, soothes ulcers, helps diabetic conditions, rejuvenates the skin, provides contentment to the heart.

3. Prepare for your fast in advance, enjoy your fast, feel younger when you end it by following the reported easy methods.

4. The Waerland System of Renewed Youth Through Fasting helped thousands of this Swedish doctor's followers. It is easy to follow.

5. Feel mental youthfulness, as did the doctor who enjoyed a controlled fasting.

10

HORMONES: KEY TO HEALTHFUL GLANDS FOR ZESTFUL LIVING

How are your glands today? If this question were asked more frequently, most folks would be healthier and happier. In order to benefit from the laws of abundantly healthful living, the endocrine-hormone network requires a Bio-Nature Health Rhythm. The body, mind, personality are all vividly influenced by a smooth-working function of this valuable glandular system.

HAPPY GLANDS: KEY TO YOUTH-ENERGY. A noted physician-endocrinologist has stated, "It is a fact that the selection of a diet has infinitely more to do with the physical and psychical make-up of an individual than has ever before been recognized. And one of the principal reasons for this is *the influence on the glands* controlling growth, stamina, energy, expression, virility and longevity."

HORMONES INFLUENCE HEALTHY PERSONALITY. The same physician-endocrinologist affirms that you can take it for granted that your thyroid, pituitary and sex glands have exerted potent influences in shaping your personality. They are closely involved with growth and nutrition; our personalities grow, too, and need good nourishment.

Personality defects are quite conspicuous in marked cases of thyroid and pituitary deficiency, leading to mental sluggishness, lack of spark and animation. Coupled with sex-gland deficiency, the consequence is a personality—or, if you wish, a "biochemical oddity"—that is difficult indeed to love as a human being.

Hormones Extend Youth and Life

A reported case is that of Mrs. R. who was in her early 60's and steadily declining in health. She had very severe generalized hardening of the arteries, high blood pressure and a scarcely discernible heartbeat. She was in a semi-coma when she was treated by the physician in the hospital. Mrs. R. was so sick, she was given up for lost.

Hormone-Nutrient Plan Restores Health. The endocrinologist who treated Mrs. R. administered an iodine supplement together with Vitamin B-complex in the form of brewer's yeast. These two nutrients were given to Mrs. R. just three times daily. It took close to 14 days before her eyelids fluttered, her skin color was firm, her breathing more regular and her pressure more normalized. This Hormone-Nutrient Plan was reportedly the only medication given to Mrs. R., yet it worked to the degree that she could soon get out of bed, go about her daily tasks, begin living again.

Mrs. R. Enjoys Life Extension Through Natural Means. After she was released from the hospital (where she had been taken as a last and hopeless resort), Mrs. R. continued taking the iodine-Vitamin B complex combination every single day. It reportedly sparked the metabolic processes to improved levels. Her hardening of the arteries now eased up, her heart was youthful, her skin had a healthy color, her personality was vivacious and she felt young all over again. Mrs. R. had more than 20 years of life added on (she reached the upper 80's) because of hormone feeding through this natural program. Glands had actually been fed through the iodine-Vitamin B complex capsule and reversed the aging process.

How Your Glands Create Healthy Living

The Health Benefit of Glands. A gland is a body organ that manufactures a liquid substance that it secretes from its cells. Some glands, such as the ductless or endocrine glands, do not secrete their liquids but leave them to be picked up and sent to other body parts by the bloodstream.

How Hormones Promote Youth Prolongation. The liquid substance secreted by the glands is called a hormone. It is known that hormones exert influence over almost all mental and physical activities. The word "hormone" is derived from the Greek *hormaein,* which means "to excite." The tiniest amount of a hormone has the power to influence growth and activity, development, tissue nutrition, sexual function, muscular tone, resistance to fatigue. Emotional and physical health regulate hormonal production,

The Body's Glandular Network. The body has eight glands forming the "interlocking directorate" of your system. These are the ductless glands, which pour their powerful hormones (chemical messengers) directly into the bloodstream. Each gland has its own function but all are guided by the master gland—the pituitary. And all of these glands need nourishment to create "happy hormones."

The Pituitary Gland

Where Located: The size of a pea, the pituitary is located at the base of the brain, directly behind the nose.

Hormone Produced: It secretes 12 different hormones including ACTH, gonadotropin, pancreatropin, among others.

Health-Producing Benefits: A healthy pituitary is responsible for the transformation, expenditure and conversion of body energy into healthful, youthful vitailty. It also produces normal sex characteristics.

Nature's Warning Symptoms: A malnourished pituitary may cause premature aging or loss of youthful enthusiasm. There may be a brain starvation which causes an abnormal craving for sweets. Directly above this gland is the hypothalamus, the appetite-sleep control center of the body. This is influenced and "fed" by the pituitary so poor appetite and insomnia may be traced to glandular starvation. A serious imbalance may cause gross overweight.

Natural Law for Pituitary Health: Protein foods such as

soybeans, lean meat, natural, organic cheeses, nuts, are especially beneficial as pituitary food. The gland tissues require Vitamins A and C found in yellow vegetables, fresh raw fruits and vegetables, carrots, fresh raw fruit and vegetable juices, too. Often, powdered protein supplements mixed with fresh fruit juice become an excellent and natural pituitary tonic.

The Thyroid Gland

Where Located: Located in your neck, directly in front of the windpipe.

Hormone Produced: It secretes thyroxine, a hormone that is formed by iodine, combining with an amino acid (digested protein) in the gland and aided by still another amino acid. In combination, these two nutrients then carry the thyroxine hormone via the bloodstream to all body parts.

Health-Producing Benefits: A healthy thyroid regulates normal growth, influences the burning (metabolization) of foods, shapes the personality and emotions and has some relation to fertility.

Nature's Warning Symptoms: A malnourished thyroid may cause abnormal weight gain, slow the heartbeat which, in turn, results in poor circulation, unhealthy skin and hair and generally deteriorating physical well-being. Some symptoms include lifeless, dry and splitting hair as well as coarse or chapped skin. Faulty elimination, senility, lowered body metabolism may also be noted.

Natural Law for Thyroid Health: The body has about 25 milligrams of iodine; this mineral is food for the thyroid. But in stress situations, the thyroid needs more iodine to issue more of its hormone. To feed the thyroid, Nature has created a powerhouse of natural iodine. It is known as *kelp.* This is a form of dried seaweed, harvested from the ocean depths, prepared in a powder form to be used in place of salt. Kelp is a mineral-rich source of food for the thyroid. It is available at most natural health food shops in powder or capsule form.

How a Store Manager Boosts His Energy. Harold E. is frequently under much stress as a manager of a large growing store. He follows many natural laws and enjoys good health, but there are times when he is nervous, irritated and emotionally unstable. To help feed his thyroid, which influences the energy-emotional balance, he takes one kelp tablet each lunchtime. He reports that this helps him maintain a tranquil outlook in the midst of stress and that he has a youthful energy. He is feeding his thyroid!

The Adrenal Glands

Where Located: There are two adrenal glands; shaped like Brazil nuts, they sit astride each kidney.

Hormone Produced: These glands secrete adrenaline, called the "emergency hormone," influential upon the autonomic nervous system. They also secrete cortin, a hormone complex including cortisone, hydrocortisone and aldosterone.

Health-Producing Benefits: Basically, the adrenal hormones control the salt and water balance in the body, use of carbohydrate, fat and protein; maintain resistance to stress, such as heat, cold, poisons; also influence muscular efficiency, reduce inflammation and allergy. In time of danger or emotional stress, extra adrenaline is released into the bloodstream where it quickens the heartbeat, increases the energy-yielding sugar in the blood, slows up or stops digestion, sluices blood into the big muscles, dilates the pupils of the eye and may even cause the hair to stand on end. All this prepares the body to meet emergency—by fight or flight!

Nature's Warning Symptoms: Premature physical exhaustion and nervous upsets are often traced to malfunctioning adrenals; allergy may be traced to undernourished adrenals, too. There may be unsightly skin lines, dark and sallow aging spots. Prolonged gland-starvation may lead to chronic fatigue, poor appetite, low blood pressure, weak pulse. This valuable gland issues its hormones to neutralize toxic waste infections in the bloodstream and a deficiency may cause sensitivity to many health allergies.

Natural Low for Adrenal Health: Among many nutrients, it is reported the pantothenic acid (a member of the B-complex vitamin group) is able to feed the adrenals and create a natural and healthful balance. This nutrient is found in nuts, seeds, soybeans, whole grains and also in raw, fresh fruits. The soybean is reported to be a powerhouse of pantothenic acid that helps nourish the valuable adrenal glands.

The Pancreas

Where Located: This narrow gland lies across the back of the upper abdomen.

Hormone Produced: The largest part of the pancreas is glandular tissue that secretes the hormone insulin and digestive enzymes and releases them by way of a duct into the upper intestine.

Health-Producing Benefits: The hormone, insulin, aids in the storage of sugar in the liver to be used for future energy needs. Insulin is the "spark" that ignites the flame to burn sugars and starches and transform them into body heat and energy.

Nature's Warning Symptoms: Without insulin, sugar, the basic source of nerve and grain energy, cannot be stored or assimilated and is finally turned to fat or excreted. A prolonged deficiency may lead to diabetes, extreme fatigue, weakness, dizziness and obesity. Advance warning symptoms include brittle nails, poor teeth, sore and bleeding gums, lip and tongue fissures and cracks, unsightly skin ailments, excessive mouth dryness, eyelid irritation, frequent urination, excessive weight loss, headaches, giddiness, nervous irritability and a numb and tingly feeling in the extremities.

Natural Law for Pancreas Health: A team of physicians at a leading hospital was able to strengthen pancreas power through natural means. They gave subjects such vitamins as the B-complex group, as well as Vitamin C. These vitamins are also found in whole grain foods, liver, soybeans, fresh raw fruits. The benefit here is that these nutrients decreased the disorder of poor carbohydrate management and glandular malfunctioning. In natural foods, the nutrients help strengthen the power of the pancreas. This team of Nature-minded physicians told patients to eliminate these artificial foods: all high-starch foods, all foods containing refined white sugar and bleached white flour, and caffeine coffee. This meant elimination of candy, cake, chewing gum, pastries, soft drinks, white bread, noodles, spaghetti, macaroni. In their place, whole grain and natural foods! It is reported that diabetes was controlled in most patients and some cures eventually occurred. The key to health was in nourishing the pancreas through natural foods.

The Parathyroids

Where Located: On the surface of the thyroid gland, in the neck. These are four glands, actually, but so tiny they can hardly be seen. Yet they have a powerful influence on health.

Hormone Produced: They secrete parathormone, a hormone that regulates the metabolism of blood-and bone-building minerals such as calcium and phosphorus.

Health-Producing Benefits: This hormone sees that calcium is stored in the long bones; it will "order" the storage depot in the long bones to release some calcium when needed to help you respond to important nerve impulses.

Nature's Warning Symptoms: Bone fragility, tetany (cramps and convulsions) and severe calcium deficiency. This means the person feels nervous irritation, poor heartbeat, irregular appetite and hair loss, visual disorders and hearing decline. The kidneys suffer if calcium metabolism goes haywire because of impaired function of the parathyroids. Since these glands influence the delicate balance of calcium-phosphorus, the body's health becomes upset; caution is the watchword.

Natural Law for Parathyroid Health: A highly concentrated source of calcium and phosphorus (the food needed by the parathyroid gland) is found in a food called *bone meal.* Here is a powerhouse of minerals. It is available in capsule form or in a delicious cooking flour that you use in place of regular flour in any recipe. It is sold at most health food and special diet shops. Calcium is also abundant in dairy products as well as in soybeans and foods containing soybeans.

The Female Ovaries

Where Located: The ovaries are about the size of olives and are situated one on each side of the womb, in the lower abdomen.

Hormone Produced: They secrete the life-giving hormones estrogen and progesterone.

Health-Producing Benefits: These two hormones offer these health building rewards:

1. *Estrogen.* This hormone stimulates the growth of the female reproductive organs and the breasts. It regulates skeletal growth, sensitizes the muscle of the uterus to pitocin (hormone) from the posterior pituitary and is a primer for the action of its twin-sister hormone, progesterone.

2. *Progesterone.* This hormone is secreted by the corpus luteum that forms after an egg cell leaves an ovary. It is essential to female fertility, preparing the lining of the uterus for implantation of the fertilized egg cells.

Nature's Warning Symptoms: Weak hormone deficiency may lead to female sterility, miscarriages, a flat-chested figure. There is a gradual weakening of health and a decline in vitality. Many women in middle years may note a form of aging that may be directly related to hormone insufficiency. In particular, nervous disorders of middle years may be traced to this hormonal slow-up.

Natural Law for Female Hormone Health: A high protein, high mineral food program is the basic foundation. Meet the onset of advancing years with inner strength and an alliance with the basic natural laws of abundantly healthful living as outlined in this book.

The Male Glands

Where Located: The male glands consist of the male's reproductive organs and the prostate gland which is located just below the bladder and encircles the urethra where it exits from the bladder. It is situated immediately in front of the rectum.

Hormone Produced: The prostate secretes a clear fluid that combines with other hormones to create male fertility. This fluid further contains substances that nourish the fragile micr-oscopic cells whose health is essential for fertility.

Health-Producing Benefits: A healthy prostate gland issues a hormone that gives vigorous tone to all body muscles, adding youthful strength to the stomach and bladder.

Nature's Warning Symptoms: Early symptoms may be a feeling of congestion, later developing into difficulty in urinat-ing. There may be little or no pain. As the gland compresses more and more, the mouth of the bladder is choked and waste passage becomes more difficult. There is an embarrassing need to make more frequent bathroom trips and a resultant feeling that the bladder has not been completely emptied. Prolonged distress may cause serious kidney obstruction.

Natural Law for Male Hormone Health: One physician reported that he treated prostate-infected males by giving them a concentrate containing an extract of alfalfa, buckwheat and soybean. Results were remarkable and in most patients, the enlarged prostate subsided. Another physician treated 19 patients with severe prostate disorder. The treatment called for elimination of all unsaturated or "hard" fats. The doctor administered unsaturated fatty acids and was able to rapidly reduce enlarged prostate in *all* 19 patients. A well-balanced and natural diet was part of the program. Unsaturated fatty acids are found in all vegetable oils!

The Thymus

Where Located: The thymus is situated in the upper part of the chest, on the windpipe and below the thyroid gland.

Hormone Produced: Called retine, it helps strengthen the body's immunity-building defenses.

Health-Producing Benefits: Retine, the thymus hormone, metabolizes calcium and phosphorus. It helps produce an abundance of white blood cells which build resistance to infection.

Nature's Warning Symptoms: A deficiency of retine, the thymus hormone, may cause a reduction in the clotting powers of the blood. Frequent nosebleeds and profuse bleeding from small bruises may be a symptom of low hormone supply.

Natural Law for Thymus Health: It is reported that the thymus gland "feeds" upon the B-complex and C vitamins as well as protein. A good source is found in whole grains and fresh fruits, as well as in soybeans, meats, fish, eggs, natural cheeses, nuts, seeds.

The Program that Helped Create Happy Glands

A physician reported that he was able to relieve and cure hormone deficiencies and glandular imbalances in many of his patients by utilizing the natural laws of healing. The basic premise is this one: *the entire body is a hormone factory. The glands are the machines that keep the body factory humming with extra healthy living. The glands are the gateway to health and happiness.*

THE HAPPY GLAND PROGRAM: The physician told his patients to reduce their intake of cooked cereals and cooked vegetables. At the same time they were to step up the use of cold-pressed vegetable oils, raw nuts, sunflower seeds, cod liver oil and unheated raw salad oils. The patients were told to *eliminate* all cooked fats and reduce starch intake. About 3 tablespoonfuls of wheat germ oil were added to their daily diet, together with whole B-complex factors derived from yeast, rice bran, wheat germ extract and liver. No smoking was allowed.

The doctor reported that when this Happy Gland Program was followed, his patients became cheerful, youthful, rejuvenated. But—when they went off the program or resumed smoking, they felt ailing and aging again.

Seven Steps to Gland Youth

The doctor prepared a list of seven steps to help regain and retain gland youth the natural way:

1. Serve foods in their original and natural state whenever possible.

2. Cook meals at low heat when possible, because high heat destroys nutrients.

3. Cook vegetables with a minimum of water, at a low heat, for as short a time as possible. Save water for other cooking uses. It is rich in gland-feeding nutrients.

4. Eat protein foods to build body tissues.

5. Avoid the use of refined carbohydrates. Use 100 percent whole grain products.

6. Avoid the use of all sugar and sweetened foods with sugar. Use natural sweeteners such as honey.

7. Emphasize nutritional value first and calories second when meal planning.

In Summary:

1. The body's glands and hormones are influential in maintaining youth, health, vitality and abundant happiness.

2. Some glands respond to specific foods but all of them require a healthful and natural diet. The seven-step "gland youth" program is easy, inexpensive and healthfully rewarding.

11

HOW TO USE NATURE'S LAWS TO BUILD IMMUNITY AGAINST ALLERGIES

Stella W. knew the misery of a stuffed nose, constant sniffling, throat-hacking coughs, as far back as she could remember. Her handbag was always amply supplied with tissues and patent medicines. Her medical budget was always strained. Stella W. would joke that she just worked to support her chronic allergies. She was so sensitive to dust and air particles that she would break out in a sneezing fit in the slightest breeze. Added to her discomfort was her loneliness. Stella W. not only looked unhealthy but she also looked contagious! She was rarely invited to social gatherings or any affairs because of her reddened nose, running eyes, annoying coughs. She was well on her way to living in isolated loneliness. Medicines were draining her budget as well as her health!

THE CORRECTIVE FOOD PROGRAM THAT RESTORED NATURAL IMMUNITY. It was through the help of a natural health enthusiast who stopped by her desk in the office where she worked as a secretary, that Stella W. found new life through an allergy-free health restoration. He told her of his own wife who was always catching one allergic ailment after another. She had developed asthmatic problems and a steadily increasing condition of bronchitis. The wife had tried prescription and patent medicines which suppressed the symptoms but did not strike at the cause of the allergies! The wife was well on her way to becoming a lifetime "medicine addict" until she began researching allergies and the building of natural resistance. That was when she found a doctor-approved corrective food program that turned the tide and caused the cessation of symptoms and eventual ending of the allergies. The husband then gave Stella W. the entire program as it was used by his wife and by the team of physicians who were able to cure their patients the natural way.

ELIMINATION OF ARTIFICIAL CARBOHYDRATE FOODS HELPED WASH OUT BLOODSTREAM. The physicians told their patients to eliminate all products made from bleached wheat or grains; i.e., white flour breads, pies, pastries, cookies, etc. *No* commercial tea, coffee or alcoholic beverages. In this diet, the carbohydrates of bleached artificial foods could be eliminated from the system and there could be created a blood-washing sensation of sparkling cleanliness.

BASIC DIET FOR BUILDING IMMUNITY TO ALLERGIES. The basic corrective eating plan called for two large vegetable portions or a vegetable and fruit salad every single day. The raw vegetable salad was the main course of the meal.

Fresh Juices. Daily, six ounces or one glass of tomato juice. Eight glasses of water were prescribed daily.

General Corrective Diet: The allergic patients were told to eat as much fresh fruit as they could daily. *No* fried foods. *No* condiments. Butter was to be added freely to all cooked vegetables and eaten generally very freely. Each day, two to four egg yolks for each adult and one to two for a child. The patient was not to hurry while eating, not to become tired or worried. He was to take a short rest after every meal.

FOODS RECOMMENDED UNDER ALLERGY-IMMUNITY PROGRAM:

Cereals: whole grain rice, corn, tapioca, rye.

Meats: lamb, chicken.

Vegetables; lettuce, spinach, carrots, squash, asparagus, peas, artichokes, tomatoes, string beans, beets, celery.

Fruits: lemons, pears, pineapples, apricots, prunes, plums, peaches, grapefruit.

Dairy Products: butter, cream, milk, cottage cheese, egg yolks.

FORBIDDEN FOODS: All artificially created or prepared foods and high-starch foods such as cookies, cakes, doughnuts, spaghetti, macaroni.

BENEFIT OF THIS LOW-CARBOHYDRATE IMMUNITY PROGRAM. The doctors reported that all of their chronically allergic patients improved clinically. There was greater resistance to offending dust, irritants and other substances that would trigger off an allergic or asthmatic or even "winter cold" spell. The benefit is that the blood becomes purified and sparkling clean under this all-natural food program. The doctors reported that whenever a patient returned to an excess of artificial carbohydrates (from bleached grain food products), there was a recurrence of allergic symptoms.

STELLA WINS FREEDOM FROM ALLERGIES. Stella W. tried this program and followed it so rigidly that she soon threw away her costly medicines and was free from allergies. But, growing overconfident, she violated the natural laws of abundantly healthful living, returned to her bleached, heavy carbohydrate foods and soon she developed such a severe asthmatic attack that she required hospitalization. It is hoped this costly and painful lesson will teach Stella W. that Nature offers hope and health for obeying her laws. There is no compromise with Nature.

How Dry Heat and Chilling Cause Allergies

Most people catch colds and develop year-long allergies because their homes are too hot instead of too cold. Central heating has turned most American homes into modified bakehouses where the air is so dry that floorboards shrink! Imagine, then, what becomes of the delicate nose and throat tissues that must have moisture to remain healthy. The dry air you breathe inside an overly heated and dry house does not contain enough moisture to keep nose and throat membranes healthfully moist. As they dry out, the thirsty tissues are more and more susceptible to allergic substances and cold germs.

HOW A LARGE COMPANY USED NATURE TO WIN THE COLD WAR! Chronic absenteeism in a large Wisconsin company called for immediate action to be taken. Since the most common cause of absenteeism was the common cold, several corrective and all-natural methods were used. It was found that this brand new sprawling insulated building was so well-built, not a bit of air could enter through any cracks. This kept the dry heat inside and it also was responsible for lack of moisture which led to cold-catching. Here is what the company did:

1. Large flat pans of water were placed beneath several radiators throughout the building's offices. That is, there was one large pan of water beneath an average working area for a dozen people. This was constantly being replaced. (The steam heat will dry these pans out which gives you an idea of how dry steam air can be.)

2. For extra-dry areas, a kettle of water was placed atop a small burner and kept boiling at low heat. The benefit here is that this released considerable steam which helped provide much-needed moisture for breathing.

3. Ordinary house plants were placed throughout the building for decorative and health purposes. The benefit here is that well-watered house plants also help raise humidity. The plant leaves give off moisture.

HEALTHFUL CONSEQUENCES. By using these all-natural methods, the company was able to build the employees' resistance to dry nasal and throat membranes and also help build resistance against chronic cold-catching. Those who followed a natural food program further enjoyed freedom from allergies. It was a reward for obeying a natural law.

PROPER VENTILATION BENEFITS WITH AN "AIR BATH." Arnold E., a lecturer, always dreaded the winter season. It meant that he would have to speak in closed-tight rooms with no ventilation. Invariably, he developed allergic attacks and winter ailments. He had to cancel many of his public speaking engagements because of this recurring ill health. His manager suggested that he accept a speaking date with the provision that the auditorium or lecture hall have proper ventilation such as an open window or draft-free air exchange. With this stipulation, ventilation would assure Arnold E. a healthful environment. This helped do the trick and his sniffles, coughs and asthmatic-like symptoms subsided. But Arnold E. loved his bleached flour pastries and white breads and his high carbohydrate intake meant only partial health restoration. Some people just never learn!

HOW PROPER VENTILATION BUILDS ALLERGIC-IMMUNITY. Generally speaking, the stuffy air of classrooms, social rooms and business establishments is to be blamed for allergic distress. Indoors, an accumulation of infectious carbon monoxide, dust and poisonous air infects the tissues of the body and renders the body vulnerable to allergic distress. Proper ventilation calls for a free exchange of oxygen from the outside to help drive out allergy-causing indoor contaminants. It is like taking an "air bath" to live in and work in a room with proper ventilation.

Four Natural Laws for "Washing Out" Allergies

A sudden change from hot to cold (both internal and external) will react upon the sensitive blood vessels in the breathing apparatus, rendering them more delicate and prone to an allergic attack. Here are several all-natural laws to help "wash out" allergies:

1. When going out into the cold air, cover your nasal passages by holding a handkerchief to your nose. This "filters" cold air so it will be soothingly mild and warm as it is breathed in. Avoid sudden or extreme temperature changes.

2. Bath water should *always* be lukewarm—or hot, if you prefer. *Never* use cold water; this means that cold swimming pools or ocean waters should also be avoided. The shock of cold water will lower your body metabolism and temperature, creating more sensitivity to allergens.

3. All foods (liquids and solids) should be warm or at room temperature. Ice-cold drinks constrict the sensitive arterial structures of the naso-pharyngeal and bronchial areas, making them overly sensitive. An allergic attack is often triggered when the system is shocked by cold drinks. In particular, avoid all soft drinks, carbonated sweetened beverages, ice creams, foods with refined white sugars and refined flours, coffee, chocolates

and other sweets. These are all rich in artificial sugar which is destructive to health-building B-complex and Vitamin C nutrients needed to feed the millions of miles of your body blood vessels.

4. Stay away from foods and beverages which have triggered your symptoms in the past. Hot spicy foods, alcohol, smoking cause not only sneezing, but itching and hives as well, in some situations. Sneeze while shaving or putting on makeup? Change your brand of toiletries. Use only bland cosmetics and shaving preparations for a while, at least. Be careful not to accidentally sniff up a noseful of powder. Even ordinary substances can be mildly irritating.

AVOID SHARP CONDIMENTS FOR HEALTH BUILDUP. Pepper, salt, ketchup, mustard, vinegar and all foods containing these sharp condiments should be eliminated in order to permit the body to fortify itself with allergy-fighting powers. By their harsh effect on the system, they over-sensitize delicate and fragile blood vessels and nasal arterial structures. Ever notice how hot you feel after eating foods that have been artificially seasoned? This causes your temperature to rise, then plummet as you cool off. This seesaw shift plays havoc with your blood pressure and figures in an allergic symptom. By avoiding highly seasoned foods, your body has the ability to fight off allergens.

WARM HANDS AND FEET ADD UP TO ALLERGY RELIEF. The hands and feet should be kept comfortably warm. If these body parts feel cold, it means there is a heavy congestion of blood elsewhere, usually in the region of the chest and brain. This unnatural blood congestion is often a precursor of an allergy attack. To draw blood away from other parts, to evenly distribute the blood, soak both hands and feet in a tub of very hot water. (Be careful that it does not burn.) Gradually, as you soak, the heat will help draw blood back to your hands and feet, warming them, re-distributing the nourishing flow and helping to render the entire body less susceptible to allergic distress.

A SWISS ALL-NATURAL HEALER FOR ALLERGIES. The hardy Swiss rely upon a folk healer for colds and other allergic disturbances. It is the *allium cepa,* according to the Latin. We know this all-natural healer as the *onion.* The Swiss have this folk remedy:

Cut a slice from a fresh, raw onion and immerse it quickly in a glass of boiled water. Do not let it remain in the water for more than two or three seconds. Throughout the day, sip the water. The Swiss reportedly use this folk remedy with remarkable success and freedom from prolonged colds or allergies.

Swiss Onion Inhaler: The Swiss also use an onion inhaler to ease stuffed nasal passages. To do this, cut an onion in half. Breathe the smell whenever you feel nasal-choked. The Swiss will keep the onion half by his bedside so he will breathe in the smell during his sleep.

Swiss Onion Benefits: The Swiss still derive further benefits from the humble but effective onion. For stiff or aching neck or congested throat, the Swiss wraps an onion half in a cloth and bandages it around the aching portion, letting it remain for a comfortably long time. This reportedly helps ease sore throat distress.

HOW CORRECTIVE FOODS CAN RELIEVE SINUS DISTRESS. Ned O., an electrician, had to work outdoors in all sorts of inclement weather. He lost many valuable workdays because a slight chill or temperature change would bring on his sinus distress. Medication only made him feel "dopey" and prone to dizzy spells from side effects. He tried diet only after he was threatened with the loss of his job and was told by a health practitioner that food could make or break one's health.

The Simple Corrective Food Program: Ned O. based his program on that of natural food. He eliminated *all* artificial carbohydrate sources. This meant he gave up all foods such as bread, cakes, puddings, pies, pastries, desserts that contained bleached white flour and white sugar. He substituted cooked fruits and vegetables with raw items. He drank lots of fresh fruit and vegetable juices. It took six weeks before Ned O. enjoyed freedom from sinus distress. And it took two weeks for him to become bedridden with a severe sinus attack—his consequence after going *off* the simple corrective food program. Now his road back to recovery is long and costly.

Benefit of a Low-Carbohydrate Program: For the sinus-stricken, a low-carbohydrate program has unique benefits. Bleached flour foods cause the bloodstream and tissues to become saturated with a highly toxic acidic waste from faulty metabolism and oxidation of excess carbohydrates and hydrocarbons.

Compare it to the turning of a wick on an old kerosene lamp. Turned on too high, the wick carries more oil than the supply of oxygen is able to burn. The lamp chimney shows a dirty black carbon residue. The same sort of situation develops in your body, except that the residue is a thick acidic waste that turns into "food" for infectious allergy-caused viruses.

Elimination of artificial foods means enabling the bloodstream to wash off its accumulated toxic agents and excessively acid accumulated plaques. Raw, fresh fruits and vegetables serve to wash off the acidic toxic waste in the bloodstream, tissues and lymphatics. A low-carbohydrate program helps the body to keep its residues down to a minimum and simultaneously ease allergic distress.

A NATURAL INHALANT. Oily nose drops or commercial inhalants do not relieve upper respiratory distress. Oily nose solutions that gradually accumulate in the nose may even cause lipoid pneumonia. One natural inhalant is *tincture of benzoin* or *eucalyptus oil* added to steaming hot water. Breathe in to relieve the feeling of fullness in the head and to soothe the irritated membranes. These two natural oils are available at most pharmacies or herbalists.

A SALT-FREE PROGRAM MAY OFFER FREEDOM FROM ALLERGIES. Many physicians report that salt is often a villain in allergic distress. The violation of the natural law here is that sodium in sodium chloride (salt) replaces calcium in the mucous membranes and tissues. A deficiency of calcium leads to the problem of dry tissues and inactive cilia, which are vital in the control of infectious organisms that trigger off allergic distress. By eliminating salt, resistance is built and immunity is increased toward allergies. This also means elimination of foods containing salt such as prepared foods. Instead of salt, look into herbal seasonings and natural vegetized salt-substitutes. These are sold in many supermarket and health food shop outlets.

Simple Exercises to "Air Wash" the Lungs

Allergies may be relieved through proper "air washing" of the lungs by means of simple exercises. It is reported that this all-natural program helped provide relief for many allergics who had been addicted to life-time medication with dizzy side effects. In this program, the allergic is asked to breathe *only* through the nose and not the mouth. Here are the three reported exercises to "air wash" the lungs:

1. In standing position, lift the heels as high as possible and lower them to the floor, both within one second. Repeat 50 to 60 times.

2. Draw in the abdominal wall and push it out again (like a belly dance) all within the space of one second. Repeat 50 to 60 times.

3. In a sitting position the sucking in of air is to be done after the allergic has mastered the preceding exercises.

Benefit of "Air Wash" Exercises: When you exhale, the chest is lowered and becomes narrower. The abdominal muscles contract. The abdominal contents are pressed against the diaphragm, elevating it from its position when you are inhaling. You should accompany this exhalation with a long-drawn "humming" sound. In the short pause after you have exhaled, the contracted abdominal muscles relax, the abdominal wall falls forward, the pressure inside the abdomen is lowered, making it possible for you to begin to exhale again. This is an "air wash" that helps refresh and invigorate the lungs.

Oriental Air-Wash Exercise: The hardy Yoga devotees find this to be most beneficial in washing out the lungs. Sit down with your elbows on your thighs, near the knees. Support your chin with one hand. Put the other hand on the stomach. Now do a "belly dance" by pulling in on your stomach muscles, then letting them relax outward, then pulling them in again. Continue for as long as it is comfortable to wash out the insides and cleanse the lungs. The natural benefit is to be able to wash out the accumulation of sludge and dust plaques that contribute to allergic sensitivity.

General Benefit of Exercises: Doing the simple exercises while standing causes the blood to flow from the head (where it forms congested allergic symptoms) to the muscles that are being active. Doing the "belly dance" exercises clears the nasal passages by redistributing the blood. Exercises will be more beneficial if performed when the person is *free* from any allergic attack. Avoid tight belts or constricting clothing. Humming as you exhale is beneficial, for X-ray studies show that it markedly improves the act of exhalation and facilitates cleansing the lungs.

REVITALIZE INNER HEALTH-SOURCES FOR ALLER-GIC RELIEF. Nature has created vital inner sources that help stimulate health and resistance to allergic distress. By utilizing the all-natural programs, you are able to strengthen and revitalize the inner sources to resist the ravages of unnecessary ill health. The goal should be the utilization of all basic natural laws, rather than just a single method, in order to reap the benefits of health, happiness and youth prolongation.

In Review of this Chapter

1. Build allergy-immunity through natural means. Eliminate artificial carbohydrate foods to help build a sparkling fresh bloodstream.

2. Irritating dry heat may be moistened with pans of water and house plants.

3. Proper ventilation helps wash out the dirt-laden lungs.

4. To help "wash out" allergies, follow the four natural laws of abundantly healthful living.

5. The Swiss all-natural healer, the onion, is reportedly successful in easing nasal congestion and providing drugless relief for choked passages.

6. Three simple exercises help cleanse the clogged respiratory system. Easy. Beneficial. Rewards? Abundantly healthful living and freedom from colds and allergies.

12

HOW TO MELT DAILY TENSIONS FOR MORE RELAXED HEALTHFUL LIVING

It is a natural law that happiness and youthful vitality rely upon the body's built-in fountain of joy. This particular fountain is known as the thyroid gland and its gushing stream of joy is the thyroxin hormone. So powerful is this one outstanding gland that malfunctioning may be responsible for laziness, emotional disorder, premature and unnecessary senility, nervous upset and so-called temperamental behavior. The power of the magic thyroid is so great that it is able to revitalize the entire personality and benefit with a feeling of joy and happiness. To activate the thyroid, several natural laws need to be followed. These include an all-natural food that has reportedly been able to awaken and supercharge a sluggish thyroid into its magic rejuventaion of the body and mind.

How a Healthy "Magic Thyroid" Can Stimulate a New-Youth

Location of Magic Thyroid Gland. This is a two-part endocrine gland that looks like a butterfly; it rests against the front of the windpipe.

Youth Hormone of Magic Thyroid. It secretes an important youth hormone, *thyroxin,* that has the all-valuable function of regulating the way the body uses its food, the rate of metabolism, or the rate at which food is broken down and built into cells and tissues. *Thyroxin* is such a powerful "youth hormone" that it stimulates the body's use of blood-building minerals and internal-feeding vitamins and amino acids.

How This Youth Hormone Benefits Natural Health. When released into the bloodstream, thyroxin determines growth, regulates metabolism, influences emotions and personality. This youth hormone vividly influences such processes as puberty, pregnancy, childbirth and the middle year conditions. Furthermore, this youth hormone is involved with other body hormones to create overall health.

The Magic Thyroid Determines Basic Health. Through thyroxin, the youth hormone, this magic thyroid influences the heart beat, the body's reactions to heat and cold, the function of memory. The interaction of the thyroid and the adrenal glands influences the blood pressure. It is known that nearly everything you do is determined in one way or another by the health of the thyroid. This gland influences health, personality, happiness, mentality, appearance.

NATURE'S WARNING SYMPTOMS OF HYPER-THYROIDISM. If the thyroid gland is *overactive,* secreting an excess of its hormone, Nature provides warning signals such as these: loss of weight, rapid pulse and breathing; goiter, eye bulging, extreme nervousness.

NATURE'S WARNING SYMPTOMS OF HYPO-THYROIDISM. If the thyroid gland is *underactive,* with a deficiency of its hormone, Nature provides these warning signals: the body's natural regulatory balance is upset and the person puts on excess weight; his heart beats more slowly which results in poor circulation; skin, hair and nails become unhealthy. The person has faulty memory and may have anemia. He usually feels cold when all others are comfortably warm. In more severe cases of a shortage of thyroxine, the person develops premature aging. Youngsters have been seen to grow withered and aged because of a malfunctioning thyroid gland. Small wonder that the thyroid's hormone is regarded as the "youth hormone."

How Youth Was Restored Through Feeding of Magic Thyroid

Youth Hormone Melts Depression. A reported case is that of Mary T., age 54. She was severely depressed and suffered from numerous phobias, especially the fear of going out alone. In addition, she suffered from chronic headaches, was overly irritable, had insomnia. Minor problems in her household were magnified until they seemed immense. She went into the hospital where it was felt that her severe depression and emotional fits could best be treated at a mental institution. Mary T. might have languished away for the rest of her life in such an institution, had it not been for the efforts of a physician who used natural means of stimulating her thyroid. Mary T. was given a thyroid-booster food, plus B-complex vitamins and a Vitamin C food supplement with each meal. She required this all-natural treatment for close to a year. Then she was able to leave the hospital, obtain a job and begin to live again. Eventually, she was discharged as being perfectly happy and normal. Mary T. had found new life through the magic power of an activated thyroid gland.

How "Youth Hormone" Added Life to a Man's Years. John R. was 36 and already had a history of three visits to mental hospitals. John R. lacked ambition, was depressed, exhausted and sleepy all the time. He was put on a natural food program and his thyroid was activated through natural means, namely, a thyroid-booster food and accompanying vitamin supplements of the B-complex and C groups. In a short time, he was able to discontinue his tranquilizers. It took close to 18 months before John R. was completely normal. He is now successful in his work and family relations. The simple and natural means of boosting the action of the magic thyroid's "youth hormone" saved his life and put youth into his years.

From Quarrels to Happy Days. Margo Y. was only 27 but she was already the victim of a malfunctioning thyroid. She had prolonged headaches, dizziness, lack of desire to work, extreme irritability, exhaustion, chest pain, backache. She was a terror to live with. She would quarrel with her family and neighbors. Only out of desperation and to avoid going to a mental hospital did Margo Y. appear for treatment. The treatment was drugless and consisted of stimulating her sluggish thyroid, as well as a return to more natural living practices, such as outlined in this volume. In Margo's situation, recovery was swift. Within three weeks after the daily thryoid-booster food and nutrient supplementation, she had a feeling of calmness and satisfaction with her surroundings. Even her backaches disappeared. The improvement in her temperament was confirmed by friends and family. It is hoped that she will continue her natural foods and the thyroid-booster eating program so as to enjoy life with joy and happiness and freedom from tension.

Emotional Upset Responds to Youth Hofmone. Henry E. was 46, and a building superintendent doing very conscientious work, when he began to feel nervous. It was not long before Henry was filled with worries as to whether or not he was doing his job right. Although there were no complaints, Henry felt emotionally upset. He developed headaches and pains in his joints that may have been regarded as arthritic. He had to undergo this natural treatment for just five weeks. Afterwards, it is reported that he was relaxed and more youthful and could deal easily with the responsibilities of his work. All this was accomplished by natural living through all-natural food boosters.

How the Magic Thyroid Prolongs Life

A physician tells of treating a 60-year old woman who was dying of generalized hardening of the arteries. He examined her completely and noted that she had an underactive thyroid gland. Because this was an emergency, the doctor administered a dose of thyroxine mixed with brewer's yeast to the dying 60-year-old woman. He continued this medication throughout the day, and then the week. The response was so great that the lady continued to use the thyroxine-brewer's yeast formula for another 20 years which were added to her life. The magic thyroid had prolonged her years.

To Have Young Arteries, Feed Yourself the Youth Hormone. It is reported that there is a decisive relationship between the health and youth of the arteries and the thyroid. It is believed that hardening of the arteries occurs when a metabolism failure permits cholesterol to collect in the arteries, instead of using or expelling it from the body. Since the thyroid gland is largely concerned with metabolism, a lack of thyroxine may be responsible for the inefficient utilization of fat metabolism which, in turn, leads to heart problems in many instances. To have smooth, slick arteries, feed your magic thyroid.

How Youth Hormone Rejuvenates the Heart. More evidence on the value of the thyroid gland to cholesterol in the blood comes from a leading university medical school. Three researchers report that cholesterol in heart patients can be effectively lowered by stimulating the thyroid gland, without stimulating an ailing heart. It is believed that people with sluggish thyroid glands do not produce enough thyroxine, the "youth hormone" which is needed to regulate the way the body uses cholesterol. Through the use of a thyroid booster food, which does not increase the heart rate, the cholesterol level is able to be lowered and the patients given a new lease on life.

The Natural Food that Feeds the "Magic Thyroid"

It is a natural law that the body's nutritional needs be met by a natural food source. The thyroid gland requires food, just as all other body parts require food. One major food is the mineral *iodine*. This mineral stimulates the thyroid and enters into the composition of its "youth hormone" known as thyroxine. Iodine may well be regarded as the spark to ignite and normally regulate a healthful thyroid gland, the key to bubbling youth and health.

How Iodine Feeds the Gland. Iodine, a mineral found in some natural foods, is ingested and then absorbed chiefly from the small intestine. It eventually enters the thyroid gland where it becomes freely exchangeable with the blood and other extra cellular spaces of the body. Iodine, when concentrated in the thyroid gland, binds with protein where an enzymatic process will facilitate its metabolization and use.

Natural Sources of Iodine

Iodine, the mineral that feeds the thyroid and enters into the composition of the "youth hormone" thyroxine, is found in foods that are grown in or near the sea. One powerful and all-natural source of iodine is *kelp.* This is a form of dehydrated seaweed. Since the plants and creatures of the sea are rich in minerals because they get their nourishment from the sea, which abounds in them, *kelp* is one powerful source of iodine.

Kelp is available in most health food stores in the form of sea salt or capsules. Use powdered or dried kelp in the manner of seasoning; capsules may be taken daily or with each meal. Kelp may well be the most powerful source of iodine that is available for the thyroid.

OTHER FOOD SOURCES FOR THE THYROID. Among other iodine-food sources, there are asparagus, dried beans, spinach, Swiss chard and most sea foods, especially haddock and flounder. If you add fish to your diet, be sure to emphasize salt water fish for they are less prone to contamination by chemicals that find their way, or are poured, into the lakes and rivers.

Several other reportedly good sources of food for the thyroid include agar-agar, eggs, fish liver oils, fish roe, Irish moss, leafy vegetables, mushrooms, salmon, watercress. Iodine is especially abundant in those parts of plants where the green coloring is most intense. Young green leaves contain more than matured leaves; stems have more than roots and the greener the leaves, the more iodine content.

Gloom-Chasing Cocktail

To help transform tension into creative energy, the thyroid gland needs normal function. Here is a simple cocktail that is able to provide a supercharging effect upon a sluggish thyroid and help put a smile in the stomach!

Steam equal portions of asparagus and spinach in vegetable oil. Squeeze through cheesecloth or strainer and drink *all* the juice. For an extra boost, add two tablespoons of cod liver oil, stir vigorously. Drink this Gloom-Chasing Cocktail in the early afternoon, each day.

KELP IS SPICE FOR THE THYROID. The miracle sea salt, a powerhouse of iodine, *kelp,* is well known for stimulating the thyroid. If there is one food that helps the health of the thyroid, it is kelp. It may be used as a spice wherever a salt is required. To further replenish the iodine resources of the body, kelp may be taken in handy capsules. Health food stores have kelp as a sea salt and capsule. It may well be regarded as the spice that is needed for the life of the thyroid!

How to Eat your Way to a Happy Thyroid

The following reported eating plan is rich in natural iodine that helps feed the thyroid to issue its valuable "youth hormone." It is again affirmed that the green leafy vegetables contain the highest amount of iodine with the root vegetables next in order. Sea foods are also rich in iodine and should be eaten several times a week. Here is a simple eating program that helps put a smile in your stomach and is the secret of a happy thyroid:

Breakfast:
>   Raw fruit
>   Cooked whole grain cereal with cream and natural
>   sweetening
>   Egg (any way, except fried)
>   Whole grain toast *or* roll with butter
>   Milk *or* hot milk flavored with coffee substitute

Luncheon:
>   (Choice): Meat, fish, eggs *or* cheese
>   Cooked vegetable with butter
>   Raw salad with dressing
>   Whole grain bread with butter
>   Fresh raw fruit *or* stewed fruit
>   Milk

Dinner:
>   Meat *or* fish *(Use fish twice weekly)*

Potato with butter
Cooked vegetable with butter
Whole grain bread with butter
Simple natural dessert *or* raw fresh fruit
Milk

(An interesting point is that the iodine content of vegetables and sea foods is not appreciably altered during the process of cooking. Of course, to faciliate and boost proper assimilation through enzymatic action, raw foods are to be emphasized.)

Herbs for a Happy Thyroid

Frank E. looked to the medicines from the meadows for a natural way to feed his thyroid and stimulate the function of the youth hormone. At a herbal pharmacy, he obtained three simple herbs: golden seal, bayberry, myrrh. He prepared a special "Happy Thyroid Elixir" by mixing together one tablespoon of each of these herbs. Then he took one-half teaspoon in a cup of boiled water as a "Happy Thyroid Elixir Tea" one hour before each meal and one last time before retiring. He found that this simple and all natural herbal tea was able to stimulate his inner fountain of youth and create natural and harmonious health. Frank E. was also in harmony with the other natural laws and was rewarded with a smile in his stomach and a smile on his face!

USE NATURE TO FEED THE MAGIC THYROID FOR YOUTHFUL VITALITY. A rich harvest of natural foods from the mineral-rich sea will help provide natural nourishment to stimulate the thyroid into pouring forth its gushing stream of joy, the "youth hormone."

In Review

1. The magic thyroid with its "youth hormone" may well be the key to emotional vitality and sparkling happy health. This one gland reportedly boosts energy, creates happiness and emotional joy.

2. By boosting the action of a sluggish thyroid, doctors were

able to melt depression, add life to a man's years, change a quarrelsome woman into a happy one, strengthen mental powers.

3. The mineral iodine, in sea foods and in foods grown near the mineral-rich ocean, is a powerhouse of nutrition for the thyroid. Iodine is metabolized to become a "youth hormone" to rejuvenate body and mind the natural way. Heart and arteries become young-feeling through iodine-fed "youth hormone."

4. Iodine is available in a concentrated form in kelp, sea salt, sea foods.

5. The all-natural Gloom-Chasing Cocktail is food for the thyroid. Make it with just two vegetables and cod liver oil for a powerhouse of glandular rejuvenation.

6. Nature has prepared a powerful source of natural iodine in special herbs. Prepared in a Happy Thyroid Elixir, this herbal tea can create harmony with Nature and benefit with joyful health.

13

HOW TO HELP YOUR HEART AND ARTERIES FUNCTION FOR MORE YOUTHFUL HEALTH

Tom J. was a hard working supervisor in a machine shop. He put in long hours. He took on extra work loads and consequently took on an extra heart load. It came as little surprise when Tom J. suddenly keeled over, clutching his chest, gasping for air, right in the middle of the machine shop. He was rushed to the factory dispensary where a series of tests told the obvious truth. Tom J. had overworked and overstrained his heart to the exhaustion point. Not only that, Tom J. had neglected many natural laws of proper rest, recreation, natural foods and had "choked" his arterial structure with unhealthful and age-causing plaques of cholesterol. Now Tom J. would have to follow a program to help him regain and retain a healthy heart and arterial system. Tom J. followed some of the program, especially the low fat schedule. Yet, he only partially recovered. He still experienced knife-like pains in his chest, shortness of breath, facial discoloration and nervous trembling. Now he went on another all-natural and drugless program of "youthification" of his heart and arteries. This program, known as the Lo-Carbo Heart-Youth Food Diet is reportedly more effective than the low-fat program because of its unique ability to strengthen and invigorate the heart-artery network which helps create a feeling of youth.

Tom J. followed the Lo-Carbo Heart-Youth Food Diet and was able to correct his health imbalance, after his low-fat program offered only partial restoration. Now he was on the road to youthful recovery.

The Lo-Carbo Heart-Youth Food Diet

How a Low-Carbohydrate Program Creates Youthful Heart. Basically, heart-harmful fatty substances are formed by overeating animal fats and also from overeating carbohydrates. While reduction in animal fats will help ease the problem of heart-artery distress, it is reported that a reduction in carbohydrate foods will be even more beneficial. Many persons who reduce animal fats are tempted to substitute with carbohydrate foods and this may cause premature aging of the heart-artery network.

Carbohydrate Foods May Raise Fat Level of Blood. In the case above, Tom J. reduced animal fat from his diet but then increased his carbohydrate intake. This caused a rise in the fat or cholesterol level of his blood so that he ran the risk of another heart attack-seizure—even on a low-fat diet plan! It is believed that carbohydrate or starchy foods are converted into sugar which is then available in fair quantities to the body. Thus, the body may use the sugar for energy, rather than the fat. So the fats, which are not used, may accumulate in the blood. Even on a low-fat diet, the small amount may be stored as the body uses the excess carbohydrate-formed sugar for fuel. Eventually, the stored fat may present a health threat, as in Tom J.'s situation.

The Body Changes Carbohydrates into Fat. The body metabolism does have the ability to convert carbohydrates or starch into fat. Those who eat carbohydrate-rich diets may be unknowingly feeding themselves large amounts of fat through this conversion process—even though they are on a low-fat diet! The key to youthful heart and arteries may lie in both a low-fat and a low-carbohydrate food plan.

Health-Helping Program

A physician created the following heart-artery youth restoration Lo-Carbo Heart-Youth Food Diet. It emphasizes a healthful reduction in foods that have high amounts of fat and carbohydrates. The great benefit here is that you can enjoy your food even while you are helping your heart-health.

AVOID THESE FOODS: Sugar, soft drinks, ice cream, ices, sherbets, cakes, candies, cookies, wafers, pastries, pies, fruit juices, canned and preserved fruits, jams, jellies, marmalades, puddings, custards, syrups.

EAT THESE FOODS IN REDUCED AMOUNTS: (These contain carbohydrates in such quantities that conversion to starch in the system may unnecessarily raise the blood fat level.) Beans (dried or lima), tapioca, macaroni, rolls, crackers, corn, peas (dried or split), potatoes (white or sweet), yams, lentils, rice, spaghetti, vermicelli, noodles, breads, buns, biscuits, commercial cereals, oat preparations, rice preparations, rye preparations, wheat preparations.

EAT THESE FRUITS IN MODEST AMOUNTS: (These fruits contain much natural sugar which may be an excess for a heart-artery conscious person.) Oranges, grapefruit, peaches, honeydew, melons, cantaloupe, watermelon, apples, pears, pineapple, strawberries, blueberries, raspberries, grapes, cherries, plums.

FRESH FRUIT-EATING GUIDE: Take just *one* portion of a fresh fruit with a meal; that is, one apple or one orange. Canned fruit juices, canned fruits, dried fruits, preserved fruits, should be avoided. *Fresh* raw fruit juices may be enjoyed in modest amounts. Fruits may be stewed but *without* sugar. Apples may be baked *without* sugar. Tomato juice is allowed since it contains no natural sugar.

EAT THESE FOODS IN UNLIMITED QUANTITY: Artichokes, asparagus, avocados, bamboo shoots, string beans, wax beans, soy beans, red beets, broccoli, brussels sprouts, cabbage, carrots, cauliflower, celery, Swiss chard, collards, cucumbers, eggplant, endive, beet greens, dandelion greens, turnip greens, kale, kohlrabi, leeks, lettuce, mushrooms, okra, onion, parsley, parsnips, fresh peas, peppers, pumpkins, radishes, rhubarb, rutabagas, sorrel, spinach, squash, tomatoes, turnips, watercress, pickles, horseradish, olives, capers, natural mayonnaise.

EAT THESE ANIMAL FOODS IN UNLIMITED QUAN-TITY: Beef, lamb, mutton, veal, poultry, fish. It is best to eat them fresh. Eggs may be eaten freely. All dairy products may be eaten freely.

LO-CARBO HEART-YOUTH FOOD DIET PROVIDES VALUABLE OXYGEN. The preceding food diet reportedly has one unique benefit. It provides an abundance of natural oxygen for the healthful operation of the heart. It has been shown that a cell utilizes oxygen in proportion as it utilizes sugar. But oxygen is useful to the cell only if there is some fuel to burn (oxidize) for the production of energy. This Lo-Carbo Plan reportedly provides much fuel for oxygen which is valuable for heart health. Furthermore, this particular program reduces carbohydrate but increases valuable protein with little fat increase. This benefit enables the person to eat fat and help keep his heart-artery network in a youthful condition.

LO-CARBO PLAN EASES HEART SEIZURE. Edward C. at age 13, was brought in by his mother because of two attacks of unconsciousness without severe convulsions. The first seizure occurred in school about an hour after lunch, lasted 20 minutes and was followed by spontaneous recovery. Edward had frequent attacks of smothering sensations and tightness across the chest upon exertion such as running. He responded to this Lo-Carbo Plan, with its high protein and normal fat diet. He became less nervous, had better color, gained normal weight. The attacks of chest pains gradually became infrequent, and stopped altogether after several weeks.

LO-CARBO PLAN HALTS CHEST PAINS. John F. came into the clinic because of attacks of pain in the upper abdomen and lower chest which came on during exertion. It was known that John F. was "cranky," easily angered, and that he always wanted to eat, preferably something sweet. He followed the Lo-Carbo Plan and was soon free of the attacks of chest and abdominal pain. There was marked improvement in general health with easing of his nervousness.

LO-CARBO PLAN HALTS HEADACHES AND DIZZY SPELLS. Murray R. had always been in good health, until his

60's. Then he began to get bouts of pain on exertion and during excitement. The attacks gradually increased in severity and frequency, so that they soon occurred almost daily after walking one to two blocks. The pain was described by Murray as "severe and sticking." The attacks of dizziness came on almost any time and often made him walk as though drunk!

Murray was given sedatives and dilator drugs without relief. He was put on the Lo-Carbo Plan but because he cut down on his protein foods, he had only partial help. But after he improved and followed the plan in totality, it is reported that he improved within two weeks. The heart pain became milder and occurred less often. He was able to walk greater distances. The epigastric pain disappeared after three weeks. Headaches and dizziness gradually disappeared. Toward the end, he reported complete freedom from these symptoms. He soon felt so well with no pain, he no longer had to come to the clinic. All the while, he followed the Lo-Carbo Plan.

When last seen, Murray R. said that he could walk up to eight blocks and return before feeling any pain. But—he did have some occasional chest pain and dizziness during excitement. Now it was learned that Murray ate bread, sugar and potatoes. He said that since he was feeling so well, he thought he could be more liberal with those foods. As a result, partial chest pains returned. When he eliminated those foods, he enjoyed freedom from angina pains. The Lo-Carbo Plan made him feel young and healthy again.

The Coronary-Youth Club

A team of physicians, anxious to help keep their patients in a heart-artery youth condition, prepared a special program which emphasizes a reduction of saturated fatty acids. This particular program is basically aimed at reducing the intake of fat as a means of helping to keep the heart and arteries in a youthful and resilient state of health. The physicians report that if the eating plan is low in animal fats, it helps provide coronary youth. The following special program was prepared by these physicians. While it may not be especially low in carbohydrates, it is presented since these physicians found it to be highly successful among their patients.

Benefit of Coronary Youth Program: This food plan is low in fat and also carbohydrate-reduced. It is known that fat and carbohydrates lead to manufacture of cholesterol and that an excess and unwanted amount of this yellow, waxy, porridge-like substance is deposited on the inside of blood vessels. These atherosclerotic plaques form into potentially harmful clot-creating knots. The Coronary Youth Program was highly successful among thousands who followed it, in conjunction with other basic laws for natural health.

Here is the Coronary Youth Program:

FISH, MEAT, EGGS

Fish: at least four to five times a week, for breakfast, lunch or dinner. The fat in fish is an excellent source of the polyunsaturated fatty acids needed to wash the arterial network of the body.

Poultry: eat often. It is low in fat.

Veal: eat frequently. It is a lean meat.

Beef, lamb: no more than three to four times a week. Each serving to be a maximum of four ounces of cooked meat. These meats are high in the saturated fatty acids.

Liver, heart, kidney: occasionally.

Eggs: no more than four eggs a week for adults; four to seven a week for children.

Avoid very fat meats—Bacon, sausage, corned beef, pastrami.

Select lean cuts of all meats.

Trim off all visible fat.

Keep portions moderate—four to six ounces before cooking (four ounces after cooking) is an adequate serving for any member of the family.

MILK AND MILK PRODUCTS

1. Two cups of skim milk daily for adults. The fat in whole milk is predominantly the saturated type. Therefore, whole milk is not recommended.

2. Two to four cups of milk daily for children. Two cups of their milk allowance may be whole milk. Skim milk contains all of the nutrients in whole milk, except most of the fat and Vitamin A.

3. More than four cups of milk is *not* recommended for children, even for adolescents. Some physicians may recommend larger amounts for pregnant and nursing women.

4. Cottage, pot or farmer cheese may be eaten often. It is low in fat and high in protein.

AVOID BUTTER, CREAM, ICE CREAM, CREAM CHEESE, HARD CHEESE, AND OTHER WHOLE MILK CHEESES.

VEGETABLES AND FRUITS

Vegetables daily: raw or cooked. Dark green leafy and deep yellow colored vegetables for Vitamin A (four to five times a week) such as broccoli, turnip greens and other greens, kale, spinach, carrots, pumpkin, sweet potatoes, winter squash. Potatoes and a variety of other vegetables for additional vitamins and minerals.

Fruits: daily.

Avoid cakes, pastries, doughnuts, cookies, muffins, chocolate, candy.

CORONARY-YOUTH PROGRAM HELPS MANY ENJOY LONGER LIFE. This particular program was reportedly beneficial to many thousands who reportedly were put back on the road of youth with proper food and living methods.

Youth-Building Benefit in Whole Grains

Because heart-artery youth depends upon a free-flowing supply of nutrient-carrying oxygen, one natural way to feed the body its supply of "breathing" is through whole grain foods. The benefit here is that whole grains, unbleached and all-natural, are prime sources of the valuable Vitamin E. This nutrient which is milled and bleached and devitalized out in processed foods, has a marvelous oxygen-feeding action upon the heart-artery system. It is reported to exert a mysterious but beneficial effect upon the blood vessels.

Vitamin E is available in non-processed whole grain foods, wheat germ oil, fish liver oils, soybeans and particularly in bread products that are unbleached and natural. These are found in natural food shops.

How Vitamin E Provides Air to the Heart

1. Vitamin E is a natural anti-oxidant in the body; it decreases the oxygen requirements of muscles by as much as 43 percent and helps push a vital stream of blood through the narrowed coronary artery.

2. Vitamin E seems to be a natural anti-thrombin in the human bloodstream. It is a substance that prevents clots occurring inside the vessel. This is the only safe and natural means of clot-prevention. (Medication often produces side effects.)

3. Vitamin E helps prevent excess scar tissue production and even, in some cases, is able to melt away unwanted scars.

4. Vitamin E is a dilator of blood vessels. It opens up new pathways in the damaged circulation, and bypasses blocks produced by clots and hardened arteries.

NATURAL BENEFIT OF VITAMIN E. One physician who saved thousands of heart-artery patients had this to say: "Vitamin E replaces 'rest and reassurance' with real help to the damaged, laboring heart itself. It is the key both to the prevention and treatment of all those conditions in which a lack of blood supply due to thickened or blocked blood vessels or a lack of oxygen is a factor or the whole story of the disease. As I have said, it has no rivals. No pharmacologist or internist can suggest another substance with all the properties and power of this vitamin. God made it unique and we ignore it at our peril."

It is possible to obtain Vitamin E capsules in most health food stores.

How to Eat Fat for Your Hearts Content

Gerald E. likes to eat meat with the taste of fat. He has

discovered a method known as "open broiling." He finds it is satisfying and also heart-soothing to cook meat in this method. He exposes the meat to cooking heat while the meat is supported by something which lets the renderings drip off. *Examples:* skewer cooking, rotisserie cooking, barbecue. This reduces fat content.

Gerald E. open-broils his steaks, hamburgers, most fish, poultry.

How to Oil Dried-Out Meats: Gerald E. will baste some cuts of meat that have dried out by this open broiling method; for this he uses liquid vegetable oils. This gives the taste of fat while eliminating the meat's harmful fat. He is thus able to spare his heart and arteries by using vegetable oils that put taste in open broiled meats.

How Gerald Enjoys Taboo Cold Cuts. While cold cuts and processed meats are high in saturated fats and also soaked with chemical preservatives, Gerald cannot resist them. He enjoys them by broiling cold cuts—this deliberately gets rid of excess fat. He also slices sausages or frankfurters and broils them for several minutes on eash side to render out considerable excess fat. This satisfies his taste, and is more tantalizing to watch and prepare. Of course, cold cuts and processed meats are unnatural and should be eliminated from the diet; but Gerald eats them in moderation and by the open broiling method, so he is partially safe. He would be more wholesomely safe if he eliminated them entirely!

How to be Good to the Heart

As a means of keeping a youthful heart-artery system, other basic natural laws include:

1. Maintain a normal weight. Overweight puts a drain on the heart and is conducive to overall weakening of the entire body. Keep trim and slim and be good to your heart and your lifeline!

2. Controlled exercise is helpful. Walking and modest exercises that cause deep breathing will help tone the heart and lungs and send a stream of fresh oxygen to the muscles of the body.

3. Be of good cheer and have a happy heart. Avoid stress

and you avoid high blood pressure. Never-ending tension eventually tightens the arteries, squeezes the coronary blood vessels and predisposes you to high blood pressure and heart attack. It is beneficial to take weekend vacations; time spent coutryside, fireside, oceanside or even bedside is helpful to create relaxation and heart-sparing health.

4. Smoking and drinking are heart-killers. Avoid these two unnatural stimulants and use natural foods to satisfy your taste and your basic heart-artery and overall health.

Herbs for Heart Youth

We learn from Nature and her abundance of medicines from the meadows. One time-tested folk healer is the *tansy herb* which is reportedly good for palpitation in the region of the heart. Make into a tea by using one heaping teaspoonful to a cup of boiling water; take three or four times daily.

For Heart Irregularity: Herbalists suggest the following tea: take one teaspoonful each of black cohosh, scullcap, valerian, lobelia and a pinch of cayenne. Mix thoroughly. Use one heaping teaspoonful of this mixture to a cup of boiling water. Steep for 30 minutes. Drink four cups a day, one an hour before each meal and one upon retiring. You may take a swallow every two hours, or a half cupful as needed. These herbs are available at most herbal pharmacies.

Natural Laws for Heart Youth Based on Folk Healers

Here is a potpourri of factors that reportedly influence the youth of the heart-artery network:

Aluminum Utensils. It has been reported that food cooked in aluminum utensils has substances that may raise the pulse and increase rate of heartbeat. It is suggested that aluminum cookware be discarded. Cooking is reportedly more safe in stainless steel utensils or heat resistant glass, iron pots, etc.

Tall Persons. Tall persons are reportedly more prone to high blood pressure. They more often have back trouble and develop more heart distress at a younger age than the rest of the population. It is believed that it takes more work for the heart to pump the blood to the head and feet of a tall person. It is doubly important for tall persons to follow natural laws to help insure and improve better heart health.

Posture. A cramped, crimped posture seems to predispose a person to heart distress. The slouching position in ordinary easy chairs may have something to do with the appearance of atheromatous lesions (hardening of the artery) in a site usually a short distance from the origin of the left coronary vessel. Proper posture may well be helpful in keeping a youthful heart-artery network.

Constipation. It is reported that constipation often is the villain in a heart seizure. Excessive straining during bowel functioning may cause a series of circulatory changes that might trigger off an attack. Straining reportedly can initiate an extreme fluctuation in blood pressure and circulation. As a means of sparing your heart, use natural methods for establishing bowel regularity. Lots of whole grains, fibrous vegetables, juicy good fruits provide natural lubrication and regularity.

BE GOOD TO YOUR HEART—YOUR LIFE DEPENDS ON IT. By following all-natural programs, your heart and arteries enjoy contentment, cleanliness, strength. Your heart was built to last a lifetime—give it a chance!

In Review:

1. Heart-artery youth receive boost through a Lo-Carbohydrate food program.

2. Lo-Carbo Heart-Youth Food Diet reportedly provides heart-saving oxygen, eases heart seizure, halts chest pains, halts headaches and dizzy spells.

3. A special low-fat diet, prepared by a team of physicians in a Coronary-Youth program, helped prolong life and health for many thousands. This diet is completely drugless, and all-natural and tasty.

4. Whole grains provide a valuable vitamin that provides oxygen for the heart.

5. Satisfy the fat taste with "open broiling" methods.

6. Herbs reportedly help ease heart irregularity or chest pains.

7. Natural laws for heart youth include cooking in non-aluminum utensils, maintaining good posture, natural regularity, basic good health. Nature keeps you as young as your heart and arteries.

14

HOW TO USE HYDROTHERAPY AT HOME TO FLUSH AWAY YOUR ACHES AND PAINS

A noted theatrical personality once said, "A hot-and-cold shower is better than a cup of coffee to get you going in the morning." He was so right! The stimulus of hot and cold water on your skin steps up your circulation and whips fresh blood cells and vital oxygen to your brain. After a brisk rubdown with a Turkish towel you will have a ruddy glow and be ready for your day. Nature has provided water for internal lubrication and for external healing, as well. Hydrotherapy is the ancient and modern all-natural healing method for restoration of the body's own "radiators" of warmth and invigoration. By using simple water-packs, fomentations, contrast bath applications, it is reported that many common aches and pains can actually be bathed away.

HYDROTHERAPY ACTIVATES INNER CIRCULATION. Water applications help revive and rejuvenate a sluggish circulation that may be responsible for many pains such as arthritic-rheumatic stiffness, headaches, localized arm and leg pains, aching stiff joints and parts, nervous tension.

Hydrotherapy at home is able to increase the speed of circulation, liberate congestion, carry extra blood to the brain and increase its supply of oxygen and nutrition. Hydrotherapy peps up circulation to help create a good feeling, improve mental alertness and body efficiency. A time-tested folk healer, hydrotherapy is completely drugless and is in compliance with the natural law of healing through Nature.

Hot Foot Bath to Relieve Headache-Chest Pains

Benefit of Hot Foot Bath: To improve the circulation in the feet and skin and simultaneously revitalize internal organ circulation. This home hydrotherapy healer reportedly relieves headache caused by congestion of blood in the brain, relieves chest and pelvic congestion. It warms the person, helps him relax and also will ease any inflammation in the feet.

Required Items: A foot tub or another container large and deep enough for foot insertion. A five-gallon can or dishpan should be big enough. Also, a bath thermometer for testing water temperature. The temperature should range from 103° to 115° F., adjusted to comfort. In the absence of a bath thermometer, test water temperature with elbow immersion. Keep adding more hot water as is comfortable.

How to Give Hot Foot Bath: The person sits comfortably in a room that is warm and draft-free. Insert the feet in the foot tub. Cover to ankles with water at 103° F. Continue adding hot water to bring up temperature, but never over 115° F. The person's feet should be immersed from 10 to 30 minutes. The feet should show a pink color. Meanwhile, apply a cold compress to the head and renew it often. It is this contrasting application of heat to the feet and cold to the head that helps relieve congestion. When healing process is finished, pour cold water over the feet and dry them. If there is any body perspiration, the person will benefit from an alcohol rub to the entire body.

Suggestions: The hot foot bath should not be given in the presence of a blood vessel disease of arms and legs, or in conditions of diabetes. Also, be careful that addition of hot water does not burn the feet. Push feet to one side of the foot tub, pour water in at the opposite side. Use your hand to splash the water around to equalize the heat.

Fomentations for Arthritic-Like Stiff Joints

Benefit of Fomentations: To relieve aching, stiff pain in

muscles and joints and internal organs. A fomentation provides natural and drugless relief of pain in internal organs through activation of nerve health; it relieves pain in muscles and joints by stirring up a fresh blood supply which soothes inflammation. To provide a natural stimulation, give a short hot application (three to five minutes) and follow with a cold application. This helps stimulate the function of internal organs and also increases white blood cell activity. The fomentation also helps calm and relax the person and reportedly relieves a nervous spasm or knife-like twist of gnarled pain in a joint that makes bending over a tortuous experience.

Required Items: A container in which to heat water, such as a large canner or pressure cooker. At least three complete fomentations (three wet packs and three dry covers. Use material that is 50 percent cotton, 50 percent wool, and 36 by 36 inches in size.) A basin of ice water. Two Turkish towels. One or two washcloths for compresses. A bath blanket or a sheet. A clean nightgown or pajamas.

How to Give A Fomentation: Have all equipment ready. Cover the aching part with a bath towel. Apply a hot fomentation over the bath towel. Protect sensitive parts and bony prominences with extra thicknesses of towel. Let the fomentation remain over the aching part until it gets cool. Then remove. Dry the treated area well, put a fresh towel onto the aching joint and then apply another hot fomentation. Simultaneously, apply a cold compress to the head and/or neck. Change every two to four minutes. After the *third* fomentation, rub the area with a cold compress and dry it. After the entire home healing fomentation, the person may be cooled with warm alcohol or a comfortable warm tub bath. The person should be comfortable, dry and free from perspiration.

Suggestions: The length of the fomentation healer is individual. Short hot applications have a tonic effect. Long mild applications have a calming effect. Very hot intense applications relieve severe arthritic-like pain—but take care to protect the person from being burned. Be careful with elderly or thin people.

Water Healing for the Spine and Abdomen

Ella T. wanted an "instant cure" for her painful back. She preferred taking costly pills. Ella T. took prescription tranquilizers. She thought this would ease or erase her arthritic-like problems. Instead, while tranquilizers did calm the nervous system, they caused a decline in Ella's alertness. Her muscles became so sedated that it was unsafe for her to drive. She felt sleepy behind the wheel and when she had a near accident with a truck on the road, she was forced to seek a drugless way for health restoration.

Ella T. decided to try water healing as a means of easing the feeling of knot-like tightness in her spine as well as the stabbing pain in her lower back. The main benefit of this water healing is in its *drugless* application. Now Ella could feel safe when driving. She had also come to develop such dependence on tranquilizers that she felt like an addict. Water healing is all-natural and drug free. Here is how Ella T. was able to free herself from drugs and help her body become restored to pain-free health .

Benefit of Water Healing for Spine and Abdomen: It helps warm up the feet. The benefit is to draw the blood away from the whirling, active brain. A fomentation on the spine provides healing heat to the little nerve centers in the back, causing a natural blood flow and feeling of spasm-relaxation. The spinal muscles start to relax. A fomentation on the abdomen helps pull out the tension (knots in the stomach) and increase blood circulation. The heat brings extra blood to the skin, drawing it from the inner organs, relieving the internal congestion. Cold compresses to the neck and head constrict the blood vessels to ease the pounding blood flow that causes a feeling of light-headedness. This natural method helps the body stir up its own sluggish healing forces to bring about relief without drugs!

Required Items: Same materials as in preceding hot foot bath. Incidentally, if there are conditions of hardening of the arteries or diabetes, heat need not be applied to the feet. Instead, wrap the feet in a warm blanket. It is beneficial to have warm feet to provide overall healing. *Additional Items:* Washcloths or hand towels to be soaked in a basin of cold or ice water, for cold compresses on the head or neck. Wring out bath towels in boiling water and when *warm,* have ready to use. Because of rapid cooling of *warm* towels, you will need to work swiftly to make changes.

How to Give Water Applications to Spine and Abdomen: The person should lie on one fomentation placed to extend lengthwise down the spine. Place the other fomentation crosswise on the abdomen, protecting the hipbones from the heat. A cold compress on the head and neck should be changed every three minutes. Change the spinal fomentation first; then change the abdomen fomentation. *Remember:* dry the part thoroughly at each change to prevent burning. Healers suggest three fomentation changes to the spine, three to the abdomen. To complete, a complete body alcohol rub or a warm (not hot) shower or tub bath. This is a natural sedative treatment. The person should enjoy a refreshing nap or sleep afterwards.

Soothing Drugless Effect: As Ella T. learned, natural healing is drugless and soothing. The preceding water treatment has a sedative effect by drawing the blood away from the head and internal organs by natural spine-abdomen heat applications. This helps ease aching and stiffness and low back pain. Ella T. could now bend over without a sharp stab that brought tears to her eyes and a bolt of electrifying sensation to her back. She enjoyed freedom from headaches without aspirin because of the cold compresses. The benefit here is that the cold compress on the head and neck eases congestion of the blood vessels of the head, helps to maintain a soothing effect; it also eases the feeling of faintness. Ella T. obeyed a natural law of health and was rewarded with abundantly healthful living.

How the Contrast Bath Soothes Muscle Spasms

Oscar D. hurt his ankle. Within a day the swelling was so uncomfortable that he could barely slide his foot into a shoe. He took aspirins to relieve the heart-pounding pain. He applied liniment to help ease the ultra-sensitive touch and the bluish discoloration. He shrugged off any suggestion of the old-fashioned healer known as the contrast bath. He relied upon pain-killing capsules and medication that did, indeed, nullify the pain but did *not* correct the cause of his foot swelling. Oscar D. neglected the natural laws and soon had to be hospitalized for a serious infection. He realized now, when it was too late, that simple water could have kept him out of this expensive hospital. Some people never learn!

Benefit of Contrast Bath for Muscle Spasms and Swellings: Soaking an aching and/or swollen foot in hot water for four minutes helps contract the blood vessels and provides a form of improved circulation. After this four-minute hot water immersion, remove the foot and soak it in cold water up to one minute. This provides internal exercise to the blood vessels. This activity greatly increases blood flow to the swollen or aching part and, by stimulating metabolism, helps promote a natural healing. This constant change from hot to cold is a form of exercise to help revitalize and stimulate congestion in a swollen or aching arm, leg or other body part.

Required Items: Two containers large enough to allow the body part to be covered with water. A bath thermometer. Several bath towels. Cold compress. This contrast bath (hot and cold water healing) is beneficial for problems of sprain, strain, impaired circulation of veins or varicose ulcers, arthritic-like distress.

How to Give Contrast Bath to Aching or Swollen Part: The person sits in a warm room that is free from drafts. The affected part is inserted in hot water (103° F. to 110° F.) up to four minutes. Remove the part and put in cold or ice water for 30 seconds to one minute. During this 30 second to one minute cold application, increase the temperature of the hot water to keep it at the aforementioned 102° F. to 110° F. A cold compress should be applied to the neck and renewed every two or three minutes. The contrasting baths of hot and cold water should be continued for up to 8 changes, taking a total of 20 to 30 minutes for the entire process. NOTE: Always end with a cold soak *except* for arthritic pain when you should end with a hot soak. Dry thoroughly. An alcohol rub or sponge bath is soothing at the end.

How a Paraffin Bath Promotes Relief from Arthritis Distress

Benefit of Paraffin Bath: By paraffin is meant the common household substance used to cover jars of jam and jelly. To use for this natural healing, add some good grade mineral oil to commercial paraffin. Heat the mixture and use for dipping the affected part. It is beneficial because paraffin requires slow, low heat to raise it to the melting point. This quality of low specific heat makes it a beneficial natural healer because it can be applied to the body at comparatively high temperatures without damaging body tissues.

Dipping an aching or stiff arthritic-stricken hand or foot in paraffin causes increased heating of the part and of the body. Because of the increased circulation as a result of the heat, the joints of the treated parts are more easily moved; exercise and massage are more easily done and healing of the joint is encouraged.

Required Items: A proper container in which the paraffin is heated. Because paraffin is flammable, use a double boiler for heating. Take care not to spill any on the stove. A standard double boiler should accommodate five pounds of paraffin and one pint of mineral oil in proper mixture. A Taylor dairy thermometer is needed. Place a cork around the top of the thermometer to keep it floating in the paraffin mixture. Also have a bath towel, a piece of sheet plastic and a basin for receiving the used paraffin.

How to Give a Paraffin Bath to Ease Arthritic-Like Pains: Because hands are often seized with arthritic-pain, the bath is especially helpful in such situations. Wash and dry the hands thoroughly. Dip quickly into melted paraffin which has a temperature from 122° F. to 130° F. (If no thermometer is available, use the paraffin after you have removed it from the fire and allowed a slight film to form on top.) After dipping the hand quickly, allow the paraffin to form into a glove. Once the glove is begun, do *not* move fingers or wrist because this may break the glove and possibly allow burning through the cracks.

Dip the hand from six to twelve times; each time, let the paraffin harden so the glove becomes thicker. Once the glove has been formed to protect the hand, the hand can be held in the melted paraffin up to twenty minutes.

Now, remove, wrap in the plastic sheet, cover with the towel. If both hands have arthritic-distress, then treat one hand first, remove it from the paraffin bath, wrap in the plastic and the towel while the other hand is treated. The heating benefit on the first hand is prolonged by treatment to the other hand.

How to Finish Paraffin Bath: Peel off the paraffin glove and place it in the basin provided. Later add water to the glove, heat the water and paraffin together, drain off the water and return the paraffin to the double boiler. This economical care will keep the paraffin clean and usable for a long time.

How Often for Healing Benefits: Generally speaking, most folks take a daily paraffin bath; then, as relief is felt, about three times a week.

Suggestions: For folks with very poor circulation of diabetes, the time-tested procedure is to dip several times to form a glove, and remove the hand quickly and wrap it in the plastic and bath towel. This prevents the possibility of a quick burn. For others, after removal, the paraffin glove makes a good mass to knead for exercising the fingers. A paraffin bath may also be beneficial to feet and specific flexible joints such as knees, elbows, forearms, wrists. Follow the same procedure and caution tips.

How to Bathe Away a Backache

The owners of a large midwestern company became concerned over increasing absenteeism because of backaches on the part of their factory employees. They had modern assembly methods and endeavored to provide comfortable working conditions but their employees had to stand for long hours, bend over and backwards throughout the day so that recurring backaches were as costly a problem as cold-catching. Medication eased the symptoms but still did not enable the body to resist back pains.

A company supervisor, with the aid of a physiotherapist, devised a set of home water healers that helped aching back problems so that absenteeism could be reduced. Here are the two home hydrotherapy programs that help ease muscular stiffness of the low back and general backache:

1. HOT SHALLOW TUB. Let lukewarm water run into the tub to take the chill from the porcelain bottom. Slowly adjust the temperature so that water is hot but not scalding, or about 112° F. Fill up to four inches, Ease yourself in and lie on your back in the warm water. Your feet are flat against the wall above the foot end of the tub; or your heels are resting on the tub's rim if it is free-standing. Slowly inch downward toward the foot of the tub until your legs are bent more and more sharply. Your back muscles now gently relax from the heat; simultaneously, stretch from the hip-rolling action of this leg position. Remain in this position for 15 minutes. You should feel a gradual loosening of cramped back muscles and general relief.

2. HOT SHOWER AND SPINAL EXERCISE. Stand with your back toward the shower. Your legs are slightly apart. Your knees are slightly bent. Put both hands on your knees. Support you upper body part with your arms. Now, let a hot spray (comfortably hot without any risk of burning) play upon your back; at the same time, arch your lower segment. Raise first one hip, then the other, in slow succession: work your back muscles gently and smoothly while heat from the shower loosens and comforts them. Remain up to 15 minutes or until you feel a "liquid free flow" of freedom from tense and tight back.

To Complete: Dry off with a brisk rub, using a Turkish towel. Then hop into bed and go to sleep refreshed! This simple program spelled drugless healing for many absentees in the midwestern company. It may benefit with a "young back" for others who feel bent over and prematurely aged because of bad back distress. It's all *free!*

Hydrotherapy Healing Benefits in Review

1. Water application, a time-tested folk healer, helps revive and rejuvenate sluggish circulation and offer freedom from arthritic-rheumatic stiffness, headaches, localized arm and leg pains, stiff joints and tension.

2. A hot foot bath reportedly eases headache-chest pains.

3. Fomentations help relieve aching, stiff joints.

4. Spine and abdominal distress may respond to simple water applications.

5. Traditional folk healer, the contrast bath, offers soothing relief from muscle spasms.

6. The paraffin bath promotes relief from arthritic distress.

7. Two simple bathing techniques provided merciful relief for countless thousands who suffered from backache.

15

HOW TO USE "FEVERS" AS NATURE'S OWN SELF-CLEANSING HEALER

"Give me the power to produce fever and I will cure disease," said the ancient physician and father of medicine, Hippocrates. This drugless healer recognized the time-tested folk practice of washing out internal impurities through a natural self-cleansing fever.

FEVER: NATURAL LAW OF HEALTH. Fever, in itself, is *not* a disease. It is a *symptom* of increased metabolism within the body as a means of rebuilding harmonious health. It is the *cause* of the fever that requires corrective healing. Fever is part of the body's defense against an invasion of infectious microbes. It indicates that the body is speeding up its counterattack—rushing white blood cells to the site of invasion, removing the debris of germ battle (wastes) and generally speeding up its metabolism to conquer and cast off the invaders.

How Fever Helped Restore Regularity. Rose T. was the victim of the laxative merry-go-round. She would take harsh cathartics, salts, and bile powders in an effort to cause natural regularity. In due time, Rose T. had weakened her internal rhythmic processes so that they could not function without the artificial stimulus of these irritating salts, powders, "milks" or tablets. To add to Rose's distress, she suffered from chronic acid stomach. Here we can see that these drugs upset the delicate acid-alkaline balance and impaired the enzymatic processes of digestion. Now she became the victim of "sour stomach" and poured more burning ointments into her already overworked and toxic-laden digestive system.

In order to help establish a Nature bio-rhythm, she began by eliminating all artificial medication. She then increased her fresh fruit and vegetable intake. She reduced bleached flour products and carbohydrates. Rose T. then took a one-hour nightly "steam bath" at home, right in her own bathroom. She would sit in a chair while the running water in the tub heated the room and she began to perspire. This caused an outflow of toxic wastes and helped start the internal self-cleansing of her vital body organs. It took close to seven weeks of natural living and a nightly "steam bath" before she could enjoy natural regularity and freedom from drug dependence. We can only hope she will continue her natural living program to enjoy abundantly healthful living.

HOW FEVER CREATES NATURAL HEALING. As an illustration, we know that a stove works well if the ventilation is in good order. If, however, it is clogged up and the air current is insufficient, the fuel will not burn brightly and leave the minimum of ashes; instead, the fuel will smolder, produce smoke and half-burned cinders which will eventually extinguish the fire altogether through lack of air.

We can apply the same benefits to fever. The body, too, needs ventilation for natural healing; that is, *air* to keep removing the ashes (metabolic waste products) which might cause the flame to go out. The natural channels of elimination in the body are the bowels, the kidneys, the skin and the lungs. These we might compare with the grate in the stove, for through them, these ashes will leave the body. If they cannot do so on account of one or more channels being blocked up, they will accumulate inside the body and, as they consist of toxic substances which the blood is trying to throw off, will give rise to *auto-intoxication* (self-poisoning) which can create impaired health. Nature, therefore, has used fever as a means of natural cleansing and self-healing.

Five Benefits of Healing Fever

Generally, a fever is a sign that the body is healthy enough to fight it out when threatened by infection. Nature creates benefits by a natural fever, among which are these self-healers:

1. *Restores Natural Acid-Alkaline Balance.* By flushing out toxic-infected cells, Nature helps wash out excess stomach acidity by sloughing off excess hydrochloric acid. This helps create what folk healers called "natural internal antiseptic washing." It is a form of restoring a soothing acid-alkaline balance that makes for happy digestion and happy health.

2. *Helps Improve Respiration.* A feverish condition leads to fast, hard breathing. This form of hyperventilation is reportedly beneficial since it increases the output of carbonic acid in an effort to decrease blood acidity. A natural and healing fever is a form of self-ventilation.

3. *Restores Body Balance.* Removal of wastes through perspiration is the natural way to wash off dirt-laden waters and acids. By washing out through the organs of elimination, the natural body balance is restored in a natural way. It is like a chain reaction that helps create smooth unified functioning.

4. *Regularity Through Normal Elimination.* During natural fever, digestion becomes more pronounced through restoration of enzymatic function. Bowel movements become more regulated. The lower bowel, where most of the fluids are absorbed, thus holds waste products a shorter time than usual because of the increased activity of the entire gastro-intestinal tract. With less fluid absorbed, the bowel movements tend to become more liquid, further facilitating a natural elimination. Those troubled with "irregularity" would do well to look upon a natural fever as a means of helping restore intestinal vigor.

5. *Helps Soothe Tense Muscles.* One young carpenter, James B., at a youngish 46, found himself losing out on building jobs because of severe muscular cramps. When he used a lightweight power saw on a piece of lumber, he would experience an iron-manacle convulsion in his shoulder. When James B. had to bend over for a brief period, he would dread having to straighten up; the knife-like kink in his lower back would cause a piercing pain. He went the route of prescribed muscle-relaxant drugs but these caused so many side effects, including drowsiness and rash on his back, that he had to give them up. When he

heard about self-flushing of toxic wastes through fever, he tried a number of home "steam baths" and enjoyed "oiling" of his constricted muscles. Great! He could move his tense muscles and work with freedom. But he discarded other natural laws of healthful food and soon developed severe stomach acid and impaired metabolism that caused arthritic-like stiffness. When last heard of, he was being hospitalized for "nerve paralysis." James B. started out with good intentions but erred by following *one* natural law and discarding the rest. There is little compromise with Nature. Successful health is enjoyed to the same degree that one follows *all* the natural laws.

A natural fever is able to ease muscle spasms and soothe convulsions by helping to moisten the clogged tissues, arteries and muscular network. In harmony with other natural laws, the body's own self-healing forces are able to work in bio-rhythmic harmony. The chain reaction helps stimulate sluggish healing and pave the way to sparkling good health.

A Comfortable Home Steam Bath for Natural Fever Benefits

The traditional Turkish bath was always regarded healthful because it produced profuse perspiration which was akin to that of a natural fever. It is still regarded as one of the most comforting ways of washing out the insides and helping to rebuild health. To take your own home steam bath you need to begin by drinking lots of water in order to make up for that which is lost by perspiration. You may use any bathroom with free flowing hot and cold water. See that you do not sit in any drafts.

1. *Sit in home steam bath.* Let the hot water create comfortable clouds of steam in the bathroom while you sit on a chair or stool. The water temperature should be hot enough to cause a profuse flow of perspiration but it should *not* be so hot that it causes weakness or energy-loss. Regulate the faucet so the heat is comfortable.

2. *Remain in home steam bath for gradually increasing periods.* Begin with a ten- or fifteen-minute steam bath the first time. On succeeding home steam baths, increase up to thirty

minutes and then up to an hour. *Caution:* there should be *no* feeling of exhaustion or weakness. Check perspiration flow by drinking fresh cool water while in the bath. This helps internal washing and also guards against weakness. If there is a feeling of energy depletion, the water should be made cooler. You may or may not fill the tub. This depends upon yourself. You will sit on a chair, *not* in the tub.

3. *Give yourself a self-scrubbing.* After you have thoroughly perspired, change the water so that the bathroom is comfortably tepid or cool. Now, use either a Turkish towel or hand mitten and give yourself a thorough rubbing in order to remove all dead skin and debris that has been sloughed through the body pores. Go all over. Some hardy folks use a body brush. This creates a marvelous feeling of tingle and aliveness that produces a sensation of rejuvenation. As you progress from a towel to a mitten, you may be able to enjoy a special body brush. Most pharmacies have them.

4. *Finish with a pore-closing cool spray.* You complete this natural home steam bath with either a cool shower spray or a brief five-minute dunk in a tub of *comfortably cool* water. You will benefit by avoiding extremes. Many folks prefer just a few moments of a cool spray in order to close the pores of the skin the natural way.

5. *Dry, wrap, rest, rejuvenate.* Dry off with a Turkish towel. Wrap yourself in a comfortable blanket to retain body warmth. Rest in your bed. Rejuvenate throughout the night in a healthful sleep. Nature rewards her followers with zesty health and youth!

Natural Fever Created Self-Defense Against Allergies

Ella J. brought in her younger sister Jennifer because she was a lifelong victim of chronic allergies. Jennifer followed the basic natural laws of nutrition and corrective healings, but her recurring allergies throughout the year (summer rhinitis, skin breakouts, winter colds, asthmatic tendencies, respiratory disorders) prompted the taking of excessive medication.

Ella believed in self-cleansing through natural fever but

Jennifer felt that if she eliminated her drugs, she would suffer from allergic distress, especially bronchitis. The physician subjected her to a battery of tests and found that many of her distress symbols could be traced to drug reactions. It has been noted that many drugs, even the aspirin, suppress fever and thus "bottle up" the body's own ventilating system. Furthermore, Jennifer took antipyretic drugs which were supposed to reduce the fever. Actually, such drugs masked the symptoms and did not kill the invading microbes. Here was a clue to Jennifer's chronic allergic trouble.

Natural Fever Turns Tide. The health restoration program called for gradual elimination of unnecessary medication. This gave the fever its opportunity to destroy offensive bacteria and build Jennifer's resistance to harmful allergens. By then following a nightly 30-minute home steam bath, she was able to flush out the toxic sludge and help restore a natural balance. It took close to four weeks before she was able to breathe without wheezing, sleep without hacking night coughs, awaken with a youthful refreshment. It was a natural program that soon gave Jennifer the coveted freedom from drug dependence and internal health. Her allergies were a thing of the past.

Medications Frequently Suppress Fever. When illness such as stiff joints, clogged insides, chronic fatigue, allergic distress, skin rashes, coughs and colds, fail to respond to medication—or get worse, despite medication—it may be Nature's signal to look to a natural-induced fever as a means of restoring sparkling inside health. Medications reportedly will often suppress a fever and this is contrary to the natural law of a fever to help rid the body of its store of accumulated sludge. Often a natural fever can be as health-restoring as drugs purportedly promise.

Nature's Proof of Healing Fever. Have you noticed that when same part of your body becomes infected and "inflamed," it not only hurts, but it also produces a miniature fever right at the place of infection? If this little local fever does not rub out the infection, poisons mount up, eventually reaching the brain's thermostat, which then fires up the entire body to battle the problem. Here we see how Nature creates fever for the purpose of healing.

Caution for Drugs. A substance which differs chemically from normal human tissues may interfere with a natural fever. So caution is the watchword for the use of drugs.

Natural Law on Body Temperature. While a so-called normal temperature differs slightly in various body parts, it is generally felt that the normal body temperature, taken by mouth, is 98.6°F. Most physicians tend to consider a range between 97°F. and 99°F., orally, a "normal" zone. One reason is that body temperature has its ups and downs during any 24-hour period. It is lowest (97°F. or less) from 2 to 5 A.M., when you're sleeping. It jumps to perhaps 99.5°F. by the late afternoon or early evening. Also, it is likely to be a little higher after meals.

Why Nature Uses Fever for Healthful Healing. Fever is a sign that a tissue or an organ has something wrong with it. The body responds with an inflammatory reaction. In an infection, for example, the body tries to get rid of the damaged tissue. White blood cells (leucocytes) infiltrate the area and devour the damaged tissue so that it can be carried out. In the process, the white cells themselves break down and often die, releasing pyrogens (heat-producing substances) which circulate to the brain and there prod the thermostat into action. Body temperature rises and Nature uses the fever for healthful washing-out and healing processes.

During an infection, other factors may cause a rise in temperature. Fever may also be associated with an illness such as gout or liver infection; an injury or burn can send bits of damaged cells into the bloodstream to be carried to the thermostat.

Your Body Thermostat. A fever, as we see, means that Nature causes the body to produce heat faster than the body loses it. As long as this happens, body temperature will rise. The body's heating system is similar to the furnace and radiator pipes in the home. When your food (fuel) is burned, the generated heat is sent through your blood vessels (pipes). For insulation, layers of fat under the skin serve to cut down unnecessary heat loss. You constantly produce and throw off heat. When production and loss are equal, your temperature is normal.

Your body thermostat is a complex mechanism governed mainly by the involuntary part of the nervous system. The body's temperature-regulating cells are thought to be centered in the *hypothalamus,* a thumb-sized area of nerve tissue on the floor of the brain behind and above the bridge of the nose.

How Nature Causes Self-Washing. During a controlled self-caused feverish cleansing, Nature keeps the temperature at a comfortably higher level. The thermostat issues signals to all vital organs. In the motion to cool the body, blood vessels in the skin dilate to permit a better flow and simultaneous muscle relaxation. The heart is helped as nutritious blood flows through its channels with more efficiency. Damaged body cells are flushed out to make more room for healthy new cells. Gradually, when the feverish condition is eased, a cooling sensation is enjoyed; inside warmth reaches the skin and the perspiration brings about a *natural* cooling-off process that drops the temperature. It is Nature's own cycle and rhythm of health restoration.

HOW NATURAL FEVER CAN BOOST HEALTH RATIO. The natural fact that you are able to work up a fever is beneficial because it shows the body is strong enough to battle a menacing virus. A fever boosts circulation, prods the body to produce more white cells to attack bacteria and to create natural antibodies to kill the germs.

Fever Helps Hormone Production. It is reportedly believed that a natural fever and a comfortably pepped-up circulation can increase production of natural ACTH, the hormone which eases the stress placed on your body by disease. This hormone, manufactured in the pituitary gland, works upon the adrenal gland to release the hormone cortisone. ACTH has been proved useful in the treatment of arthritis and many other joint distress problems. Fever may well be a clue in the healing of arthritic-like symptoms.

HEADACHE RELIEF THROUGH FEVER. A well-known writer and public lecturer, Michael T., was the victim of recurring headaches. The nature of his work produced much eyestrain. His problem was that aspirins worsened his condition and he had attacks of migraine. Michael T. would enjoy relief through home steam baths, but his problem was that he had to travel a lot and could not follow other Natural Laws while on the road. But Michael T. reported freedom from migraine and eventual relief from pounding headaches through home steam baths.

How Natural Fever Relieved Michael's Headaches. In this fellow's situation, abrasive wastes were set loose by harmful bacteria from commercial and chemical-treated foods. These abrasive wastes entered the bloodstream; here, they would flow up to the base of the brain where a group of toxin-sensitive cells would become bunched. Alarmed by the poisons, the cells sent emergency messages to all parts of the body which help in conserving heat. As the heat outlets became closed, Michael's skin became dry. At the same time, blood vessels would contract, making him appear pale but preventing fever-heated blood from cooling off at the body's surface. This caused the pounding headaches and migraine attacks.

Michael T. relied upon Nature to induce a natural fever that would enable the germ-laden body cells to become flushed out and thereby ease the head congestion. It was this all-natural and time-tested folk healer that helped bring about relief from headaches for this writer and lecturer. His basic health would have improved even more if he could have followed other Natural Laws.

How to Help Nature in Her Healing Fever

Here are seven natural laws that help Nature provide corrective healing through a home steam bath fever:

1. The person should not be chilled as this always upsets temperature balance. Apply some form of heat to the feet to prevent chilling. This helps bring blood to the surface and allow cooling of the body.

2. Since a lot of water is lost through perspiration, and also through vaporization from the air passages, drink lots of water during the process; also enjoy fresh fruit and vegetable juices.

3. Rest is essential. It is important to get lots of good sleep each night. Daily "cat naps" are also soothing and relaxing.

4. Since a fever-like and increased temperature very quickly burns up much of the reserve of protein and essential fat and carbohydrates, the diet should include foods that have good protein and natural unsaturated fat. Carbohydrate-energy is formed through fresh fruits and natural-sugar fruits.

5. Use light bed covers and keep the bedroom comfortably cool. Sweating it out by huddling up under blankets in an overheated room is unwise. After all, the body is striving to get rid of the heat, not trying to conserve it.

6. Cool water applied to the skin absorbs heat and cools the body parts and the blood near the skin. The simple cold compress (a cloth wrung from cold water and folded to fit the part in need of soothing, such as the back of the neck during headaches), changed frequently is most soothing. Bathing of the hands and arms with cool or tepid water also reduces temperature through natural evaporation. These simple natural methods help provide much comfort during the home steam bath.

7 To benefit from a healing natural fever, *avoid* caffeine which expands the brain's blood vessels, bringing more blood to the brain. *Avoid* aspirin which suppresses or bottles up the fever, contradicting the Natural Law of releasing stored up wastes.

Healing Herbs During Fever Wash

Folklore has learned that herbs are soothing as well as healing during a fever wash.

Herbal Tea: Take 1 heaping teaspoon of *golden seal* and ½ teaspoon of *myrrh.* Steep together in a pint of boiling water for 20 minutes. After taking the first cupful, take 1 tablespoon every hour, thereafter.

Cleansing Tea: Just ½ teaspoon of *slippery elm* in a pint of water will provide a healthfully cleansing herbal tea to be taken during a home fever program.

Health Booster: Dissolve 1 tablespoon of whole wheat flakes in hot soybean milk. Sip slowly. The magic secret here is that the soybean milk is *naturally alkaline*. This helps soothe the digestive system and gives a gentle coating of comfort.

NATURAL FEVER: NATURE'S MAGIC HEALING PROCESS. Nature has seen fit to provide the body with a fever mechanism to help promote natural healing. Cooperate with this basic Natural Law and reap the benefits of abundantly healthful living.

Main Points in this Chapter

1. Fever is a natural mechanism by which the body can dispose of disease-causing wastes.

2. A home steam bath creates a feverish condition which restores acid-alklaine balance, improves respiration, establishes regularity, eases headache congestion, offers muscle-relaxation.

3. Build self-defense against allergic symptoms through a home steam bath.

4. Note the seven ways in which a corrective-fever can provide healthful healing.

5. Herbs reportedly provide soothing relaxation during a home "fever" program.

6. The Health Booster, made of two all-natural ingredients, promotes digestive joy by giving a natural gentle coating of comfort to the vital organs.

16

HOW TO USE HELIOTHERAPY (CONTROLLED SUNBATHING) FOR EXTRA HEALTH BENEFITS

How Sun Healing Corrected Aching Joints. While carrying an armload of bundles, Irma T. lost her balance and fell to the ground. A vise-like wrench twisted through her ankles and legs. Her arms felt as tight as gnarled ropes. When she was helped to her feet, walking was painful for Irma so that she had to use a delivery boy to carry her purchases home. For many months thereafter, Irma T. suffered from painful knees and elbows as well as twisting spasms whenever she bent over at the waist. Medications relieved the symptoms but when the effect wore off, the pains returned.

Unable to do housework, Irma T. closed her home and went to a resort in a sunshine region of her state. Here, she idled away the days on the sun porch because her pain-twisted limbs made movement a chore instead of a natural action. That was when Irma T. began to feel soothing relaxation. Bathed by the warm and comforting rays of the sun, her joints became tranquil and restful. After three weeks of "sun healing," Irma T. could open and close her fists without a grimace, she could bend her knees without yelping in a spasm, she could get in and out of the bathtub with flexible hip movements that were youthful. Now Irma T. could enjoy freedom from her aching joints. The warm rays of the sun had promoted a natural health restoration. But when Irma T. went back home, away from the warmth of the sun, the joint aches returned with such severity that she required hospitalization and sedation. True, Irma T. could not spend her entire lifetime in a sunshine environment, but she could have taken advantage of the natural law of "indoor heliotherapy" through sunshine-substitutes. Had she done so, she could have enjoyed freedom from joint aches.

Six Natural Laws of Heliotherapy

Healing sunshine and sunshine-substitutes offer six basic benefits of health-plus that are free for the taking. These include:

1. *Youthful Energy Through Sunshine Stimulation.* Turn yourself toward sunshine and drink in the salubrious rays as if they were dripping with sweetness. A boundless source of radiant energy can be tapped by taking a brief time to absorb the stimulation of controlled sunshine. To feel zippy again, it is unnatural to drive yourself harder until you feel that about-to-drop slump. Instead, take a few moments off to give the body a chance to catch up, to repair and rebuild resistance, to snap back. One of the finest times to do this is after lunch. If possible, eat in a quiet place in the sunshine. Sit still. Just think and be motionless. Drink in the sunshine's youthful energy. Soon, you'll feel the blood rushing to the skin surface, and a ruddy, warm glow will pervade your very being. You will feel rested, relaxed. A wonderful "it's-great-to-be-alive" feeling will replace your half-dead, dragging-your-feet slump. All this is yours when you take time to let the sunshine energize you with its radiant energy.

2. *Sunshine Is a Natural Skin Tonic.* Ultraviolet light shining on the skin provides a great natural health benefit. It is capable of manufacturing Vitamin D in the skin, which helps nourish the cells and tissues that lie beneath the surface. Sunshine increases the number and efficiency of blood vessels in the skin. You will notice that folks from Hawaii or other islands where there is plenty of sunshine have a soft, velvety-textured skin. This is because their skin has more blood circulating in it

than the skin of the average city dweller who lives indoors. The sun calls up special cells in the skin named *melanophores*. They produce a layer of pigment along the basal cells of the skin; in essence, the tanning process. These cells protect the skin from too much sun. Sunshine in controlled doses is soothing, softening and beneficial to the skin. Certain skin disorders such as acne, psoriasis and infection are cleared up by controlled sunshine. Old Sol can well be considered a natural skin tonic.

3. *How Sunshine Can Be a Blood Circulation Tonic.* When Arthur R. shook hands, it gave the feeling of a cold fish! He had sluggish blood circulation and a threat of anemia that did not respond to costly pharmaceuticals. He had become resigned to his cold hands-cold feet discomfort and sickly pallor, when a co-worker ridiculed him about his "clammy hands" and his "cold fish face." This made Arthur R. so self-conscious that he developed a nervous eye twitch. It was this chronic and embarrassing twitch that sent him to a physician who believed in utilizing natural laws of healing wherever possible. He suggested sunshine as a tonic to boost circulation and thereby send a stream of warm oxygen-carrying blood cells to his extremities. Arthur R. tried indoor and outdoor heliotherapy and was able to balance his circulation and warm his hands and put a healthy glow on his face. This calmed his nerves and relaxed his twitch. But the problem here is that Arthur R. went back to his indoor life with hardly any outdoor sunshine exposure; he grew overly confident and soon became so anemic that he needed expensive injections to help build up his sluggish blood circulation. Now his hands and feet felt like ice; he shivered even in the warmth of his room. He had strayed from the natural law of sunshine for blood-boosting and was paying the unhappy penalty.

Heliotherapy is a healthful form of cellular-stimulation that helps bring blood to the skin surface. The ultraviolet rays of the sun help increase the white blood cell count which provides immunity from infection and health-restoration through natural means. We know that plants hidden from sunshine become pale and sickly. So it is with the person who is starved of the vital blood-building rays of the sun. These sun-starved folks are denying themselves valuable *solar energy*, the great all-natural healing force.

4. *Relax Your Way to Health Through Heliotherapy.* Sunlight is a great relaxer, for what is more soothing than sitting on a park bench in the sunshine and taking the luxury bath of Old Sol? The warmth of the sun brings a relaxed tingle and glow to your body after the winter cold and indoor confinement. A noted physician suggests, "As soon as the sun is out, do not waste coffee breaks on a drugstore stool but take a stroll in the park or sit on a bench and soak up the healing sun. You will find it relaxing, and as soothing to the nerves as a chemical tranquilizer." Sunshine exposure on the golf course or while you walk in the park or down a country road is great fun and a wonderful way to relax. As the skin imbibes more of the sun's rays, it stores up enormous amounts of inner energy. The sun provides one of the most natural remedies for the nervous person who is filled with anxiety, worry, frustration, stresses and strains. When these tense people enjoy sunshine, its soothing rays give them what their nerves cry out for: *relaxation.* The benefit here is that as you bask in the warm sunshine, millions of tense nerve endings absorb the magic ingredient of sunshine—*solar energy*—and nourish the nervous system of the body. Heliotherapy and solar energy become a tonic, a stimulant and above all, a GREAT NATURAL HEALER.

5. *How Sunshine Helps Clean Out Infectious Germs.* The natural law here is that the rays of the sun are miraculous germicides. The benefit is that sunshine causes a pale, anemic, lusterless, toneless skin to become smooth, soft, rosy and resilient. Sunshine raises the resistance of the skin so it can more quickly dissolve and cast off the infectious germs that threaten abundant health. Sunshine builds up the blood by helping to increase the red blood cells and pep up the white blood cells. The red blood cells act as the carriers of food and oxygen. But white blood cells *kill germs* and all infectious wastes, so sunshine is needed to stimulate the production of many more of these white blood cells, so essential as self-cleanser. Someone considered sunshine as "an ointment in healing up wounds and better than any salve man made" because it

has the power to kill germs and stimulate natural healing. Another vital benefit is that when sunlight causes increased circulation to the skin, this in turn flushes out the impurities from vital internal organs—liver, lungs, kidneys, skin pores. Self-cleansing is a natural law that is fulfilled through controlled sunbathing.

6. *Oil Stiff Joints with Sunshine Healing.* Creaky joints with arthritic-like symptoms are the bane of more and more folks. It is a natural law that ultraviolet light shining on the skin is able to manufacture Vitamin D. This nutrient plays a decisive role in the metabolism of calcium and phosphorus; it is known that in conditions of stiff and aching joints, there is an imbalance and deficiency of these two minerals. Sunshine, through activation of Vitamin D, is able to create an "oil can" reaction by providing calcium and phosphorus to lubricate and provide flexibility to stiff body parts. This was noted in many hospitals where patients with gnarled and twisted joints were wheeled out into the sunshine to absorb its healing benefits and help establish mineral balance so that twisted body parts could become resilient and youthful again. Sunshine may well be regarded as Nature's magic health tonic!

Ancient Folk Healing for Modern Times

Heliotherapy, an ancient folk healer, is slowly becoming recognized as a modern method for miracle health benefit. Sunshine healing is one of the oldest known means of treatment, its history going back to the days of the sun worshippers who believed that all life stemmed from the sun. They prayed to the sun for health, and also exposed themselves to the healing rays of sunlight.

Greek Method of Natural Healing. The famous Greek physician, Hippocrates, knew of the benefits of sunshine healing. He created special "sun parlors" or solariums in which health-seekers could enjoy the warmth of the sunshine for healing. The word *solarium*, which we use today to designate a room in which the body is exposed to sunlight or artificial light, is taken from the Latin word for *sun*.

Swiss Discovery of Ancient Health Law. A Swiss healer, Arnold Richi, was the first of a modern group to revive the ancient health law of heliotherapy. Later, two Swiss physicians, Dr. Bernhard and Dr. Rollier, reported healing many patients with sunshine. As far back as 1910, they called for light healing and sunshine for health. Dr. Rollier is often called the "father of modern heliotherapy." He coined the word "heliotherapy" from two separate Greek words which, taken together, mean "sun treatment." Sanitariums in Switzerland emphasized heliotherapy as a basic natural law for overall healing.

How Healing Is Created Through Heliotherapy. The Swiss healers learned that controlled sunshine is able to stimulate the blood circulation, accelerate sluggish reactions, revive circulation and ease painful symptoms, Sunshine rays have a unique benefit in that they become absorbed by the protoplasm (the body fluid containing most vital elements needed by the body). This absorption results in physical and biological healing in the body. Thus, healing is stimulated through sunshine.

How to Benefit from Sun Healing

To protect the body and skin from excessive burning, it is best to wear sunglasses, a hat to shield scalp from harsh exposure, and to apply protective lotions to the skin. Since the sun is the strongest between the hours of 11:00 A.M. and 2:00 P.M., it is best to keep out of the open during those hours to avoid over-exposure. Most heliotherapists suggest gradual exposure to acclimate the body to the outdoors.

The first day, there should be only ten minutes of exposure; the second day, 20 minutes; then the third day, about a half hour. Slowly, as the skin becomes tanned, the person exposes more and more of himself. Always wear a hat to protect the head from direct rays of the sun.

Select a Clear Environment. Edna R. took precautions to avoid sunburn. But she erred by thinking she could enjoy sunshine in a region that was drenched with smog. So she wasted her efforts, experienced little health restoration and was more discouraged than ever. The reason for her failure is that the rays of the sun vary at different altitudes because of the dust, smoke and moisture in the air. It is noted that heliotherapy is best applied at high altitudes; if at low altitudes, it must be in a clear environment, an area that is dry and free from the dust and smoke found in the air over city areas. Edna R. should have discussed her plans with a physician and also a travel agent who could have guided her on an appropriate location for healthful sunshine.

Natural Law of the Air Bath. Since Louis T. must care for his ailing wife, he is rarely able to get to a region where sunshine could provide healing for his taut nerves and his pale skin. But Louis T. knows of another natural law—that of the air bath. He lives in a mountain region that has some sunshine, but not enough. Therefore, Louis T. does the best next thing. He exposes his body to the cool mountain air. The benefit here is that it has a powerful natural tonic reaction, accustoms his sickish skin to the soothing and healthful air. This helps relax his nerves and also tones up his skin. He may go for an hour or two in the cool mountain air. While sunshine may be modest, he benefits from the natural law known as *aerotherapy*—taking an air bath. Even if he must remain with his wife and is unable to go to a sunshine resort, he obtains partial benefit from the air bath and modest sunshine exposure. Compromise where necessary but take advantage of as much of the natural law as possible.

Indoor Heliotherapy—Sunshine Substitutes

Ned E. and his wife, Doris, have a small hotel which takes much of their time. They rarely take a vacation since they cannot leave their hotel to any assistants. Ned does not trust them. His health problem is his poor circulation and he complains of feeling a heavy weight on the back of his neck. This sore shoulder stiffness is often Nature's warning of possible arthritic distress.

Ned E. and Doris once were able to escape to Florida sunshine when their married son and daughter-in-law took over the hotel for a month. This helped Ned who came back with a healthy skin glow, a springy walk, completely energized. He felt light and flexible. So did Doris. But after a short spell of constant indoor living, Ned soon felt stoop-shouldered and old His son and daughter-in-law lived in a distant state and it was rare that they could take over the hotel to permit Ned a well-earned vacation in the healing sun. Ned tried indoor sunshine. It did not work.

How to Sunbathe Through the Window. Ned lost out through indoor sunbathing because most of the sun's beneficial rays do *not* penetrate readily through window glass or thick layers of solid plastic. So Ned tried something else. He applied 5 mil polyethylene film to the outside of his screen or window frame. Now, with the window *open,* the film held in the warm room air but did not exclude sunlight. Now Ned could benefit from some ultraviolet ray warmth that this special 5 mil polyethylene film did *not* screen out (glass does screen it out), and he enjoyed partial relief from congestion. He could walk better. He followed other natural health laws of proper nutrition, rest, and natural foods, and even though he had minimal outdoor sunshine exposure, this program helped provide soothing benefit. If Ned could have enjoyed complete outdoor sunshine, he might have been able to recover fully.

The Natural Law of Healing Through Light Bulb Heat

Create a substitute form of indoor sunshine through a simple light bulb. Shield your eyes from the glare; then bake uncomfortable body parts with healing rays from an ordinary incandescent light bulb. For more direct benefits, use a metal reflector to help direct the heat toward the ailing part. If a metal reflector is unavailable, line the inside of a lamp (a plain desk lamp usually works well) with a cloth or paper shade with aluminum foil. Be *careful* not to get any of the metal in contact with the electric socket. A simple 200 watt bulb (or two 100 watt bulbs) spaced two or three feet from the aching part usually provides relief within a few moments. Move the lamps closer or farther to adjust the heat, and bake the part about 15 minutes at a time. It is reported that this indoor "sunshine substitute" with a simple bulb provides healing heat to an aching part. No sun tan, but soothing inner warmth and comfort.

Relax Muscle Tension with Body Baker Lamp

His sharp pain in the lower back region of the kidneys was first felt when Louis Y. bent over to pick up a heavy tool box in his garage. He cried out when he tried to straighten up. It caused such severe painful spasms throughout the next week that Louis Y. could not report to work for several days. Anxious to be cured, he submitted to drug injections that may have eased the spasm but caused a severe skin rash and dizziness as well as nervous tension. He was taken off the medication, but now suffered a more painful muscular spasm. He had to take more time off from his garage.

In bed, he leafed through several home mechanic magazines and came across a rather simple device that reportedly could be used to create a "body baker" lamp. It was said that "indoor sunshine" could be enjoyed with such a lamp.

Louis Y. had been told that a few months in a healthful sunshine resort could ease his muscular spasm, but he could not get up and go off that easily. So he decided to try this so-called "indoor sunshine" program with a body baker lamp.

How Louis Y. Made His Own Sunshine. A shallow wooden crate is lined with aluminum foil. Through the slats, insert a socket to which an electric light cord is attached. In the socket, screw a *luminous infrared lamp* known as a deep therapy lamp. Louis Y. then propped up the wooden crate and turned on the lamp, stretched out beneath the glow and enjoyed "indoor sunshine" for 30 minutes at a time. The warmth soothed his aching lower back to such a degree that after ten or fifteen such "indoor sunshine" sessions, he could return to his garage and work with smooth flexibility. He continued with his nightly "indoor sunshine" sessions for two more months until he felt resilient again. Heliotherapy created a miracle of healing.

Benefit of Deep Therapy Lamp. This special lamp, available in most hospital or medical supply outlets and many pharmacies, has a unique heliotherapy benefit. Its artificial sunlight provides comfort to the nerve endings that are connected between the skin and the internal organs. The artificial sunshine helps arouse the internal healing forces, relax the muscles and relieve painful congestion.

Stimulates Natural Circulation. The deep therapy lamp simulates sunshine in that it produces warmth to the blood vessels, increasing the volume and flow of blood. It draws blood congestion from internal organs and muscles; it helps evenly distribute gathered or congested blood corpuscles and send them into re-established circulation. This eases muscle spasms and provides relief such as that enjoyed by garageman Louis Y.

Wear an Ice Cap to Improve Circulation. A folk healing suggestion is that during "indoor sunshine" or even natural outdoor sunshine, the person wear an ice cap or cold towel around the head. The secret benefit here is that the cold is used to prevent cerebral anemia (drawing too much blood away from the head region) due to vasodilation (dilation of blood vessels), caused by application of heat to the rest of the body. In so doing, the head is kept cool and heliotherapy is able to concentrate on the other parts of the body. A cold towel or an old-fashioned ice cap on the head is all that is required.

How Long to Use Body Baker Lamp. To begin, the body baker lamp should be kept about two feet from the sore part being warmed. If this home healer or "indoor sunshine" is used to warm and relax a body part (muscles are relaxed by the soothing effect of the heat rays on the nerves), then just ten minutes of exposure is regarded as suitable, If deeper therapy is needed, about 30 minutes would be helpful. If there is a severe muscle-joint problem, then up to one hour may be used. It is reported that this natural "indoor sunshine" lamp is comfortably safe if there is no feeling of burning. In one specific treatment, such as for brachial neurosis (nerve inflammation of the arm), the body baker lamp can be soothing for as long as two hours.

The emphasis here is on *warmth* rather than heat. Just as warm water can be soothing while hot water can burn, so it is with a *warm* lamp that can increase oxygen, while a *hot* lamp can lead to internal congestion and scorching.

An Ounce of Prevention Is Worth a Pound of Cure. It is a natural law of health that prompt action is necessary at the very outset of discomfort. One stubborn woman, Lorraine E., refused to admit that she was "getting on" and ignored Nature's warning symptom of a slight muscular ache. She so neglected little warning symptoms that she soon developed severe and irreversible arthritis conditions. Now Lorraine E. required a cane and extensive care to ease her pains; her legs were so stiff she could scarcely bend them at the knees. So we can readily appreciate the natural law of acting promptly upon a warning symptom. In Lorraine's sad case, ignoring her symptoms turned her into an invalid in the prime of her life, dependent upon her husband and children.

How Nature Sends Warning Symptoms for Heliotherapy. Muscle and joint pain often lead to cramp-like spasm. This may cause more pain and increased abrasion on surrounding joints from too-tight musculature. A slight injury may often cause recurring aches; inflammation permits blood proteins to leak out of overexpanded blood vessels. Continued neglect creates a focal site for "muscular rheumatism" and arthritic tendency. This explains the reason why many healthy young athletes develop premature joint degeneration because they neglect simple injuries and minor alarm signals. Many such discomforts are Nature's warning symptoms for corrective health measures and utilization of the law of heliotherapy. Warmth, whether from sunshine or "indoor sunshine," could often stop the slow, insidious increase of health decline.

BENEFITS OF INDOOR LAMPS. Generally, home lamps offer benefits for problems of hyperemia (unusual amount of blood congestion in a part), provide an analgesic (pain relief) benefit. Warmth also creates an anti-spasmodic effect that relieves muscular spasms, and creates a germicidal benefit by destroying harmful germs.

The Sunshine Carbon Lamp

A well-to-do industrialist rarely has ill days, even though he is in his very late 60's. He follows the various natural laws of healing but maintains that his enviably good health comes from a *sunshine carbon lamp*. This man is able to melt nervous tensions and ease aching parts by devoting about 30 minutes to an "indoor sunbath" with this lamp. It works well for him. No secret here. Such lamps have always been used for heliotherapy.

The Miracle Sunshine Lamp. The carbon arc "sunshine" lamp consists of two carbon rods or electrodes clamped into a reflector in such fashion as to allow their free ends to come together. This carbon arc lamp is the oldest substitute source of sunshine in use today. It is available at houseware stores and special hospital or medical supply outlets. To operate, just flip the switch!

The sunshine carbons are so called because they furnish a substitute radiation that is more like that of healing sunshine than any other type of ultraviolet lamp.

How to Use: Caution is the watchword, as with open sunshine. Enjoy *slow* and *gradual* exposure. Lie beneath the lamp (about 30 inches from the body) for ten minutes at a session. Shield vital or sensitive organs and eyes from the glare, just as you would from the open sun. It is suggested that the lamp be placed at an 80° angle to minimize problem of burning.

Benefits of Sunshine Carbon Lamp. Through the deep healing penetration action of its ultraviolet rays, the sunshine carbon lamp is able to stimulate metabolism, increase mineral absorption in the marrow of the bones, help awaken hormonal flow, improve tone, color and elasticity of the skin. It also helps increase both the red and white blood cells and the bactericidal powers of the blood. Heliotherapy through "indoor sunshine" can often be as beneficial as outdoor exposure.

MAKE FRIENDS WITH SUNSHINE. Whether you bathe in sunlight or with the aid of lamps, protect your face from direct rays to prevent excess skin wrinkling. Use baby oil or vaseline as a protective coating. Work up to a gradual tan. Twenty minutes of sun or lamp exposure provides as much benefit as any larger amount with reduced risk of leathery skin or other problems which may follow extreme overindulgence in sunshine exposure. It is a natural law that moderation in all good things helps provide an abundance of healthful living! Make friends with sunshine and enjoy renewed health.

Highlights of Heliotherapy Benefits

1. Controlled sun healing offers youthful energy, improved skin health, stimulated blood circulation, cellular rejuvenation, drugless relaxation without tranquilizers, internal germicidal action, flexibility of joints.

2. Sunshine healing was used in Swiss sanatoriums where natural laws helped promote internal forces of recuperation from degenerative illnesses.

3. An air bath provides a natural tonic and helps soothe the nerves and the skin.

4. Indoor heliotherapy can be enjoyed by using a special film over an open window so that helpful rays can reach the affected body part to promote healing.

5. Ordinary light bulbs reportedly provide same healing benefits as sunshine.

6. A body baker lamp provides "indoor sunshine" to heal joint aches and spasms.

7. The sunshine carbon lamp is helpful for indoor heliotherapy. You can "make your own sunshine" with this simple lamp, available at most large appliance outlets.

17

HOW TO USE ORIENTAL BREATHING SECRETS FOR HEALTH REJUVENATION

The Oriental and Yoga practitioners of drugless healing have long recognized breathing as one of the most powerful forces of health restoration. Corrective breathing programs formed part of the rejuvenation quest by the mystical Hindus, the Tibetan lamas (holy men), the Sanskrit learned men of Indo-Europe, as well as the modern Yogi (wise men). These drugless healers felt that corrective breathing techniques and programs could relieve internal disorders, set up a chain reaction to enable the body to self-heal and self-rejuvenate. They created different types of a *mantra* (Indo-Oriental–Tibetan formula) that purportedly helped create renewed life and health as well as correction of illnesses. They realized the power of proper breathing.

Benefits of Breathing Programs

The ancients inscribed benefits of breathing programs in scrolls and parchments as well as in forerunners of our modern books. The Veda (the four holy books of the Hindu practitioners of drugless healing) contains a description of the following ten basic benefits of proper breathing. Modern Yoga-breathing draws from these ancient secrets described in the holy Veda:

How Corrective Breathing Creates New Life

1. *Dissolves poisons.* When you wash out the entire lungs with fresh oxygen, you help burn up poisons that might otherwise cause internal injury and abrasion or internal pollution.

2. *Enriches bloodstream.* Corrective breathing helps add and properly nourish millions of health-giving red blood cells in the bloodstream.

3. *Creates natural vitality.* When natural and sufficient oxygen is fed to the entire system. it helps provide a form of natural stimulation. Proper breathing is an all-natural stimulant.

4. *Bestows a light feeling of youth.* With nourishing oxygen as food for the bloodstream, there is a light feeling of buoyancy that creates a youthful sensation of vigor and health.

5. *Deep breathing is a natural purifier-healer.* The Indo-Orientals of the Himalayas long benefited from the secret that deep breathing is a natural purification source. Today, the oxygen tent in the modern hospital is able to heal when other methods are inadvisable. Regular deep breathing is an ancient natural healer that promotes vigor and strength. Even broken or brittle bones heal more quickly when the blood is nourished and purified by corrective breathing.

6. *Improve mental powers with breathing.* Deep breathing is known to help nourish the cells of the brain and thereby sweep away stagnation and sluggishness. Many nervous disorders respond favorably to proper breathing.

7. *Corrective breathing helps stimulate thinking processes.* Healthful fresh air that is sent streaming throughout the head creates stimulating vibrations. Many eye, ear, nose and throat specialists are aware of the benefit of proper aeration of regions in the head. The oxygen sent by the air waves into the regions of the eye, ear, nose and throat is able to sweep out germs that are lodged therein and helps restore a stimulating circulation to these parts. Thinking becomes more acute and invigorated through proper internal ventilation.

8. *Improve circulation with corrective breathing.* Many who have problems with cold hands, cold feet, cold noses and

ears would do well to help improve circulation with proper breathing. Sufficient oxygen is able to improve circulation. It is a Hindu natural law that the more oxygen in the system, the better and more efficient is the circulation.

9. *Put tone into the muscle with proper breathing.* Flabby muscles and wrinkled skin often respond to fresh oxygenation. The muscles have a natural tone. The skin is firm and youthful.

10. *Internal massage through fresh air exercises.* Corrective breathing creates a natural internal massage of diaphragm stimulation. This gentle and all-natural internal massage is able to improve digestion which is the key to abundantly healthful living.

Three-Minute "Brain Alert" Breathing Exercise

The scrolls of the Tibetans have a special three-minute "Brain Alert" breathing exercise that helps promote mental stimulation. It's simple, easy, effective. *Here's how:*

Stop what you are now doing. Sit up straight. Put both hands on your hips and hold them firm. Take a series of deep breaths. Hold each breath for the count of five. Exhale. Continue for three minutes. Then return to your work.

Benefit: The Tibetans knew that many people feel tired, sluggish and mentally fatigued because they do not supply their brains with enough oxygen through deep breathing. The preceding Oriental exercise is beneficial because it sends a fresh supply of oxygen whisking through the lungs into the bloodstream and thence, carried by the red cells, to the brain This helps "alert" the brain, wash out toxic wastes and invigorate the thinking processes. The brilliant philosophy and mystic knowledge of the Tibetans have never been surpassed. Small wonder that they reached such intellectual heights when they knew the super-charging brain powers of simple breathing.

How Breathing Creates Super-Brain Power

Because breathing is so common, so "every-dayish," it is taken for granted and abused. Yet, when this natural force is marshalled and utilized, it has the power to create super-brain ability. The Orientals knew that ordinary breathing sustains life; but corrective breathing improves and strengthens the body and mind. Their legendary wisdom and spiritual heights attest to their super-brain powers through corrective breathing.

How Oxygen Is Food for the Body. The lungs are the pipes of the body. The lungs need food—oxygen. The lungs have about 750 million air sacs, or cells, through which the oxygen passes to get into the bloodstream. If we could stretch these tiny air sacs from one pair of average lungs onto a flat surface, they would cover an area of 455 square feet. Yet each air sac must have its food—oxygen.

The Bloodstream Is Nourished by Oxygen. At any given second, one quarter of the blood in the body (an average person has about six quarts of blood) passes over the surface area of the lungs to give up the carbon dioxide gas that it is carrying. The blood then takes oxygen from the air we breathe for the return circuit to the cells.

The Cells Transport Oxygen to the Brain. The cells transport this oxygen-food to all body parts, especially to the brain. These are the red blood cells (about 250 million for every *drop* of blood). So strenuous is the work performed by these cells that each one lives only about 30 days. This means that 12 million cells must be produced every second of every day; all this to provide oxygen to the millions upon millions of cells throughout the body.

The Cells Influence Brain Power. The Orientals and Hindu super-brain geniuses may not have known our modern physiology, but they knew that the cells which carry oxygen could either improve or deplete brain power. Today we know that the cells which react most to oxygen starvation are *the brain cells*! So the most essential benefit of corrective breathing is to the brain! Without a good, clear brain and stable emotions, there is loss of control of the very essence of life.

How Breathing Creates Natural Brain Generation. The Brain is the electric dynamo of the body. Medical science can actually measure its electric current. Where does this electricity come from? How does the brain receive its electric power and enjoy self-generation? One basic source is through oxygen! Healthful oxygen breathed into the lungs and circulated in the blood-stream helps create a generation power to electrify the brain and the entire system.

Nature's Warning Symptoms of Faulty Breathing. Improper oxygen means that the higher centers of the brain are first affected. Nature sends warning symptoms such as impairment of reasoning, will power and judgment. So-called senility may often be traced to an oxygen-starved brain! Every cell requires its share of oxygen that is food for the brain and the entire body—and for life itself!

Oriental Basic Breathing Law

The Basic Breathing Law, taken from the Hindu–Oriental-Yoga discoveries, calls for these three simple practices:

1. Stand erect, feet slightly apart, back of hands together down in front of you. Inhale while lifting hands overhead. Separate them. Spread them to the sides level with your shoulders. Now exhale and relax while bringing hands to the original position.

2. While walking, or in any position, force air out in short breaths through pursed lips in a "shush" or whistle a tune of some kind, and inhale in short sniffs, forcibly snuffing in through the nose. This Hindu-inspired breathing exercise helps flush out internal debris through exhaled air.

3. Close one nostril with your fingers. Breathe in, in sniffs, through the other nostril. Now close this nostril, exhale and then breathe in the same way through the other. Alternate up to ten times. This Yogi exercise helps clear the nasal passages and relieve symptoms of sinus-like congestion.

The Morning Energizer Oxygen Cocktail

Paul N., a somewhat sluggish clerk at a paper mill, found himself dozing off in the early hours of his job. Paul admitted to losing other jobs because he was such a "slow starter" and would waste half the day in just "getting started." He might have lost this job except that a co-worker asked him to attend a

Yogi class one evening, and that was where Paul N. heard of a special Morning Energizer Oxygen Cocktail that worked wonders for "sluggish brains." He practiced the demonstration in the Yogi class and then he began to practice this four-step corrective breathing program at home, every single morning, when he awakened:

1. In the open air, or with windows open, Paul stood with hands on his lower ribs.

2. Paul breathed in slowly through his nostrils; he had to be sure that his *lower* ribs were being pushed out. (Many people breathe without using the lower rib muscles to their fullest capacity and thereby deprive their brain cells of the full force of oxygen food.) Paul had to practice to accomplish this second step.

3. At the end of breathing *in* (inspiration), after taking in all the air possible, Paul took in another whiff. Then he took one more. As he took his last whiff, he hooked his fingers under his ribs and gave them a gentle tug outward.

4. Now, with his mouth open, he let all the air out; at the end of this expiration, he pushed the lower ribs *in*. He grunted to get the last bit of air out. He repeated this Morning Energizer Oxygen Cocktail up to ten times. He found it swept out cobwebs, flushed out sluggish cells and gave him the start he needed. Paul N. was now able to get to work on time and was able to hold onto his job.

Natural Breathing Laws for Respiratory Healing

Florence T. was a lifelong victim of bronchitis. She had tried medication which brought relief for her symptoms, but which did more than help her wheezing, air-hungry plight. They many persons who have respiratory ailments, when the basic cause is untreated, it grows steadily worse and develops into asthmatic problems. Many who develop emphysema (known to be the largest increasing killer in America) were original victims of bronchial disorders, which insidious respiratory ailment kept increasing until it developed into a fatal form of emphysema. So we can understand why Florence T. wanted to be cured of her bronchial distress.

A Middle-of-the-Night Coughing Spell. Awakened in the middle of the night with a hacking coughing spell, Florence thought she would suffocate. When she turned all shades of purplish-blue and almost collapsed, she was rushed to the hospital. Here she underwent a series of breathing exercises that did more than help her wheezing, air-hungry plight. They started her on the road to cure. She has always been grateful for that middle-of-the-night threat of suffocation and her hospital breathing programs.

The problem of the asthmatic or respiratory-distressed person is *not* to get air into the lungs, but rather to get air *out* of the lungs after it is in. Spasm of the tiny tubes in the air sacs may be caused by an allergy or some other factor. Prolonged oxygen imbalance may cause the lung to lose some of its elastic quality, making the job of getting air out of the lung even harder. In the following hospital-supervised program that restored Florence's health, one benefit is to be stressed.

Corrective Breathing Is Required as Part of Natural Law. While proper breathing exercises help ward off bronchial attacks, and will help control and cure, it is essential that these programs become a part of the natural law of healing. If exercise is not regularly and faithfully done, the person is not benefited, just as medicine on the shelf does not help the person for whom it was prescribed. Fit these SIX LAWS OF RESPIRATORY HEALING into your daily program.

NATURAL LAW 1—RELAXATION. To stimulate self-healing forces, relaxation is essential. You may begin, as did Florence T., by lying on your back, knees bent. *Relax!!* Put hands lightly on the upper abdomen. Now, since the benefit is to get air *out of,* not into the lungs, after you have relaxed, the emphasis is on exhaling.

Exhale slowly, with the *S* sound. The goal is to make the *S* sound as long as possible without taking in a new breath. The upper part of the abdomen is relaxed afterward, then a normal breath is taken and a short rest is allowed. After the rest, a normal breath is taken, and the exercise is repeated. After ten such expirations, permit a long rest period of quiet breathing.

NATURAL LAW 2—LOW-RIB BREATHING EXERCISE.

Florence sat in a relaxed position in a chair. A belt was placed around her low ribs. She grasped the ends which were crossed in front, one in each hand. She exhaled slowly, allowing the upper chest to empty, then the lower chest. She finally drew gently on the two ends of the belt to assist in emptying the base of her lungs. She expanded the low ribs against the belt and breathed in quietly. She kept her arms and shoulders *relaxed* during exhalation until it was time to pull on the belt.

NATURAL LAW 3—POSTURE HELPS BREATHING. Good posture helps improve aeration of the lungs. In standing, tuck the hips well under, keep the abdomen flat, the knees slightly relaxed. Let the body weight rest on the balls of the feet. Proper pelvic positioning brings the other body parts into line so that the shoulders and head are in good position.

How Proper Sitting Benefits Oxygen Flow. When sitting, sit well back in a chair that gives good support, with the feet supported on the floor. Proper sitting posture gives the chest ample opportunity to expand. Slouching cramps the lungs and prevents oxygen flow and impairs inner ventilation, especially of the lower chest where respiratory distress is strongest. So Florence improved her sitting posture and gave her lungs a chance to breathe fully!

NATURAL LAW 4—STRAIGHT-LEG RAISING. Florence stretched out on her back; a small pillow under her head. She began by keeping her knee straight, raising her leg from the floor or bed until it reached a 45° angle. She repeated this with the other leg. She would *exhale* as she raised her leg; she would *inhale* as she lowered her leg. She did this slowly to permit adequate oxygenation-breathing, both in and out.

NATURAL LAW 5—HEAD AND SHOULDER RAISING. Still lying on her back, Florence raised her head and shoulders off the floor or bed. She would *exhale* as she raised up; she would *inhale* as she lowered herself to the starting position.

NATURAL LAW 6—BREATHING AGAINST RESIS-TANCE. In an effort to benefit with synchronization of abdominal and diaphragmatic breathing, Florence had a medium-sized book placed on her abdomen, just below the first ribs. The book gently rose and fell with inhalation and exhalation. It is important to get the feeling of breathing directly *under* the book, for that is where the diaphragm is. Although the diaphragm is the chief muscle of respiration, often it is neglected because of shallow breathing.

WHEN TO EXERCISE: It is suggested that the preceding set of natural laws be followed in the morning and in the evening after adequate clearing of the air passages. Florence T. was told to follow these exercises at home whenever she felt a bronchial attack coming on. She later reported that she was able to actually control or eliminate an approaching attack through proper breathing, relaxation and consciously trying to assist the air *out*. She did not return to the hospital again so it is hopefully assumed that corrective breathing helped solve her problem of bronchial distress.

Breathe Right—And Stay Well

As we see, your health is largely influenced by proper breathing. Oxygen is vital to every cell in the body. As oxygen burns food, energy is released for muscular labor and body warmth. Waste products such as uric acid are prepared for excretion by oxidation. Your blood circulation is the longest and strongest line of body defense against disease; oxygen is the purifier of the blood and helps resist infection.

Sluggish Breathing May Cause Heart Distress. Often, improper breathing is one leading cause of a stroke or coronary thrombosis. A noted physician has said that a sagging diaphragm may predispose a person to a heart attack. He explains that an insufficient supply of oxygen may slow down the heart's action. The blood flow being sluggish, a blood clot may form and plug the coronary artery, causing a heart attack. So we can readily appreciate the benefit of expanding the diaphragm and giving the bloodstream a fresh supply of life-giving oxygen.

Walk Your Way to Better Health. A brisk walk of 20 minutes means that your blood will become enriched with four times more oxygen than when you sit quietly in a chair in a room. For some folks, impaired health is the result of not getting enough blood pumped through their body each minute to eliminate waste products. With their body cells clogged and their brains foggy, their health declines. To send more oxygen through your body, take regular walks and supply your bloodstream with oxygen—the lifeline of better health.

Ten Golden Laws for "Oxygen Healing"

The Sanskrit mystics called breath or oxygen by the name of *prana*. They developed the following Ten Golden Laws that act upon the body with a vital force, as an absolute energy of energy. We can see that corrective breathing, as developed by the mystics of the Indo-Orient-Europe nations, could produce the blessings of good appearance, good health and long life.

Benefit of the Following Ten Golden Laws. The Oriental secret here is that proper breathing motion is able to recharge the body batteries and send a life-giving force of clear air surging through the lungs for overall body revitalization. It should be noted that these mystic healers relied entirely upon drugless methods for health correction. These Ten Golden Laws, drawn from their long-forgotten scrolls and mystical writings, were undoubtedly as potent as medicines in creating long life and health. Today we find that many of these exercises are being used in modern practice by medical men. The ancients were well aware of the power of these natural laws. They were well ahead of their time. We may drink from this fount of wisdom of drugless healing through corrective breathing.

BASIC POSITION. All of these breathing exercises should be done in the morning, after awakening. Stand straight. Keep feet level, ankles firm, calves tight, knees snapped back, thighs firm, buttocks firm (most important), spine straight.

GOLDEN LAW 1—LIVER AND GALL BLADDER AWAKENER. Assume the basic position. Now, inhale slowly. On the abdomen just below the breast where the liver and gall bladder are located, massage downward. Hold the breath for the count of ten, while you massage downward on the abdomen.

GOLDEN LAW 2—DIGESTION STIMULANT. Assume the basic position. Inhale slowly and hold the breath for the count of ten. While holding the breath, vigorously slap with the open hand the whole abdomen area from the rib cage to the navel. It is good to wet the hands with cold water when doing this exercise.

GOLDEN LAW 3—THE KIDNEY AND BREATHING EXERCISE. Assume the basic position. Inhale slowly. Hold the breath to the mental count of ten. Now reach in back of the body, just below the rib box, with both hands. Place a hand on each kidney. Now, while holding the breath, put gentle pressure on the kidneys and bend the body as far backward as possible. Straighten up. Repeat five times.

GOLDEN LAW 4—KIDNEY VIBRATION. Assume the basic position. Inhale slowly and hold the breath to the mental count of ten. Now, instead of putting pressure on each kidney, vigorously pat each one as you repeat the preceding motion. It is beneficial to wet the hands with cold water to get good stimulation and circulation to the kidneys.

GOLDEN LAW 5—SPINE VIBRATION. Assume the basic Position. Inhale slowly and hold the breath to the mental count of ten. Now, while holding the breath, bring the arms horizontal to the sides and slowly turn the body from left to right. It is important to keep the head facing forward and the hips locked forward; it is only the body from the waist that is moving from side to side. You should be able to twist the body five times to the left and five times to the right.

GOLDEN LAW 6—SPINE-JOINT FLEXIBILITY. This is helpful to ease the back muscles, unlock the spine and permit a flow of living energy throughout the body. Sit on the floor, raise hands over head and inhale slowly. Now, with knees straight, reach forward and touch fingers to big toes, at the same time trying to touch the forehead on knees. While doing this, slowly exhale air through mouth.

GOLDEN LAW 7—MASTER ABDOMINAL EXERCISE. Lie on floor, flat on back. Raise left foot and point toe. Inhale. Now lower left foot within one inch of floor, at the same time raising right foot to pointed position; exhale air from lungs through the mouth as the left foot goes down. Inhale as the right foot comes up. Do ten times with each foot for the first time. Increase until you can comfortably do at least 15 lifts with each leg. UNIQUE BENEFIT: This is a most unusually beneficial exercise. It is a natural stimulant for the entire abdominal region and acts as a natural vibrator. It gives the liver, gall bladder, spleen, stomach a natural jiggling. It awakens the entire digestive system and helps create youthful power.)

GOLDEN LAW 8—BACK AND SHOULDER EXERCISE. Lie flat on back, arms and hands reaching in back of you. Inhale through nose. Now bring both knees up to the chest while at the same time the arms reach down and lock the legs just below the knees; exhale the air. With all the strength of the arms and shoulders, pull the knees down on the chest. Now return the feet to the original position but do not let the heels touch the floor. Repeat five times daily. Increase until you can comfortably perform 15 times.

GOLDEN LAW 9—LEG AND ABDOMINAL AWAKENER. Lie flat on your back. Raise your heels one inch off the floor. Inhale through nose. Now, open the legs as wide as possible but keep them one inch off the floor. Exhale through the mouth as you open your legs; inhale as you close them. Keep legs straight. Do not bend knees. Repeat five times daily. Increase until you can comfortably perform 15 times.

GOLDEN LAW 10—SPINE AND SOLAR PLEXUS. Lie on the floor, face downward. Reach in back of body and clasp hands. Inhale. Now, raise head upward and backward as far as possible; at the same time, press the arms and hands downward in back of body and then exhale.

FURTHER SUGGESTIONS: The ancients suggested that a comfortable bath be taken after these breathing exercises. After the tub or shower, do *not* use a towel. Instead, use your hands and rub your legs, arms, shoulders, back, abdominal regions, with a quick, peppy rub. It may seem at first that you are never going to get dry under this procedure, but the increased circulation and body heat does the job. It also causes a natural increased respiration that washes the lungs and helps provide an overall feeling of invigoration. To complete, you may rub yourself briskly with a heavy towel. Rub until your skin is as glowing pink as you can make it. This helps create a youthful, healthy and beautiful skin that breathes life and youth!

THE BREATH OF LIFE. As we see, fresh air is your invisible food. Proper breathing causes self-healing, purification through life-giving oxygen, mental ascent, emotional ascent. To permit oxygen to flow freely, it is suggested that clothing be comfortable, *not* confining with tight constricting garters, girdles, belts, braces and the like. They choke off the free flow of oxygen. Furthermore, tight clothing causes shallow and rapid breathing, a symptom of nervous tension. To benefit from youthful energy and better body functioning, there should be unobstructed oxygen flowing through the circulatory system. It may not help you feel better *today,* but it may help you keep feeling better *tomorrow,* and better the next day and so on. When walking, standing, sitting, lying down, breathe deeply and breathe well. Your life depends upon it!

Chapter Highlights:

1. Simple and corrective breathing techniques were known to the Indo-Oriental-Tibetan mystics. They realized that proper breathing is able to dissolve poisons, enrich the bloodstream, restore youth, create healing, improve mental powers, revitalize circulation and cause internal "air massage" of vital body organs.

2. The three-minute "Brain Alert" breathing exercise is reportedly a dynamic morning energizer.

3. Flush out impurities and revitalize the brain cells with the Oriental Basic Breathing Law.

4. Start the day off with youth-power through the Morning Energizer Oxygen Cocktail.

5. Respiratory distress responds to six natural laws. They helped Florence T. correct her bronchial disorder.

6. The Sanskrit healers developed drugless healing through Ten Golden Laws for "Oxygen Healing." Simple programs help awaken the liver, gall bladder, digestion, kidneys, spine, joints, abdominal organs, back, legs and arms.

7. An "Air Wash" is a natural law that promotes self-rejuvenation and miraculous health.

18

HOW TO GET TO SLEEP REFRESHED FOR DYNAMIC HEALTH

One of the most important and basic natural laws of abundantly healthful living concerns *refreshing sleep.* A good night's sleep should be refreshing when you first go to bed and should be refreshing when you first awaken. This may well be the Great Law of super-health. All of the other natural laws will provide youth-bestowing benefits when this Great Law of sleep-refreshment is fulfilled.

THE 20-MINUTE PATTERN THAT INFLUENCES THE ENTIRE DAY. The health-happiness-success pattern of each day can be (and usually is) formed during two ten-minute periods: the last ten minutes before you sink into sleep at night, and the first ten minutes after you awaken in the morning. This Great Law is the conditioning technique that can provide health-building sleep at night and youthful momentum to carry you through the day ahead. It may well be that the Great Law of these two ten-minute periods is the most valuable of all natural laws. Once you have learned how to take advantage of these two ten-minute periods, how to turn them to your advantage, you can benefit with super-health and emotional youth. There is nothing complicated about this procedure. It calls for all-natural and drugless methods of providing the mind and the body with a healthful desire to go to sleep refreshed.

How to "Deep Breathe" Your Way to Refreshing Sleep

Charlotte T. was a bundle of nerves. She was so tense that she would lie awake half the night, staring at the ceiling, counting off the minutes in frustrated insomnia. She took prescribed sleeping pills and barbiturates but they left her drugged and dizzy and she would walk around in a daze the next day. So she eliminated them and needlessly endured health-depleting insomnia. It was during one of these stare-at-the-shadows insomniac sessions that she turned on the radio and listened to one of the all-night talk shows. The interviewed guest was a sleep specialist who explained that a simple "deep breathing" program could sweep away congestion and help provide a refreshing sleep without drugs. Charlotte listened desperately, as would any person who suffers from chronic sleeplessness.

The Deep Breathing Program for Refreshing Sleep. The radio guest outlined the simple program that Charlotte followed:

1. Breathe in and out through both sides of the nose for ten times.

2. Breathe in through both sides of the nose but breathe out through *one* side of the nose; close the other nostril with a finger. Do this for ten times.

3. Breathe in through both sides of the nose and now breathe out through the *other* side of the nose; close the first nostril with a finger. Do this for ten times.

4. All of these deep breathing exercises should be performed while lying on the back.

Natural Sleep-Inducing Benefits: This rhythmic breathing provides internal ventilation and the casting out of harsh irritants that may grate the nerves and cause insomnia. It is known that tension-causing insomnia may be a symptom of irritation of the nerve endings in the naso-pharynx region and of the reflexes generated by it. The deep breathing exercises help to melt these tensions and offer relaxation and sleep.

Ten Minutes of Deep Breathing Provides Soothing Sleep. Charlotte T. followed the exercises for ten minutes and when she felt her eyelids getting heavy, she closed them and drifted off into a light sleep. She enjoyed her sleep until early morning when the radio (she had forgotten to turn it off) came forth with a blast of loud music. Now Charlotte T. could enjoy sleep with the breathing program. But she still spent her days in fretful tension because she did not start off the day with a program of Ten Golden Minutes of preparation. But she is grateful for being able to sleep at night. She follows the Deep Breathing Exercises almost every night. If she would start off the day properly, she might enjoy better health!

Start Off the Day With Seven Natural Laws of Morning Pep

Ralph H. is an amazingly energetic and vital person who lives in a chaotic business whirl, yet is always relaxed and happy. He says he follows these seven natural laws of morning pep after he awakens. He says that you would not even start off in your car without giving it a moment to warm up, so he does not want to plunge carelessly into his day without conditioning himself for it. Ralph H. has found that when he follows these laws, he supercharges his mind and body with such youthful energy that he is able to go forth into the competitive rush-rush world with natural tranquility and bubbling vigor. This is quite a welcome contrast to those who rely upon narcotics to provide pseudo-sleep and pseudo-energy. Here is Ralph's all-natural program:

NATURAL LAW OF THE "AIR BATH." Begin each of the following Seven Natural Laws with the *basic air bath*. Stand before an open window (avoid direct drafts) and breathe deeply. Normal or habitual chest breathing is shallow and rapid; it has a one-two count of inhale-exhale. But for energy-breathing, you need to go deeper. Your intake and outake should be slow, deep and rhythmical. Your purpose is to take fewer breaths—but deeper ones. Inhale deeply to bring your lower abdominal wall into action. Let go. Relax. Pause as you let go. Now take in another *deep* and leisurely breath, feel it wash out your insides, then let go slowly. Relax. Continue ten times. Always let the air wash into your bellows. Do not force yourself. Let it come naturally. Think of the basic air bath as being smooth, like a gentle wave washing up on a shore and then quietly receding. This creates a rhythm that helps establish an *orderly pattern* that will influence the *harmony* of your day's activities.

Note, especially, the pulsations in your abdominal wall in the "V" below your rib cage. These pulsations are important since they indicate a restoration of peace and harmony and clear thinking that is essential for the success of the day ahead.

As suggested above, begin each of these seven natural laws with the basic air bath. According to Ralph H., he would not think of going forth into the hurried world of competition without first conditioning himself with self-ventilation and a "warm up." Here are the seven natural laws of self-energy that boost the energy capacity of the body and mind for the day ahead:

1. AWAKEN YOUR ARMS. Stand with both feet a dozen inches apart. On the count of "One" stretch your arms forward, upward and look up. On the count of "Two," drop your arms and head heavily, letting your chin rest on your chest. Permit hands to swing back and forth until they come to an easy halt. Repeat up to five times.

2. LUBRICATE YOUR STIFF WRISTS. Stand with hands in front of stomach, palms facing your body. Shake your wrists loosely and lazily. Continue until you have a flexible or well-lubricated up-and-down movement. Gradually drop your arms down and shake the entire arm. Repeat up to 20 times.

3. PUT A SPRING INTO YOUR LEGS. Stand and hold your balance by touching the wall or a chair. Shake your left leg. Kick and shake your hip and knee joint to benefit with a loose, flexible leg and ankle motion. Now repeat with your right leg. Repeat up to 20 times. (NOTE: This natural law is especially beneficial to those who either stand or walk on their feet a great deal. One mailman, George E., who suffered from such severe leg and knee cramps that he was almost forced to retire, followed these exercises and was able to "put a well-oiled spring" in his legs. He was able to retain his job and walk with flexibility.)

4. HOW TO LIGHTEN THE "HEAVY SHOULDER" WEIGHT. You may either stand or sit. Inhale and lift your shoulders forward and upward in an exaggerated position to try and touch your ears. Keep head normal. Let go slowly, moving shoulders backward. Now relax and drop your shoulders. Return to first position. Repeat five times. You may increase the lightening-weight feeling if you breathe in and out in a leisurely manner.

5. HOW TO PUT FLEXIBILITY IN YOUR HIPS, BACK AND ABDOMEN. Stand with feet spread about two feet apart. Toes are to be turned out 45 degrees. Now breathe in and out and let yourself relax. *Drop your torso.* Let your upper body drop down in a straight line, trunk erect. At the same time, bend your knees slightly and let your head fall forward with a jerk; rest your chin on your chest. Drop your shoulders and dangle your hands between your knees. RELAX. Breathe in and out. Return to starting position. Repeat six times.

6. THE "RAG DOLL" FEELING FOR EMOTIONAL HEALTH. The unique benefit of this simple program is to keep your spine flexible, to help provide a relaxation of the shoulders and arms that further relieves tension on the back of the neck. With this "rag doll" relaxation, you are able to think clearly and coherently and are able to face the day with confidence and healthful enthusiasm. Stand with feet two feet apart, toes turned out. Breathe in and out deeply. When you exhale or "let go," then "flop" your trunk forward at the waistline. Let your arms dangle toward the floor and your head hang limp like a rag doll. Relax. Breathe in and out. Return to starting position. Repeat five times.

7. THE HEAD CIRCLER TO STIMULATE MORNING POWER. It is reported that tight, cramped and kinked muscles felt in the back of the neck upon awakening, can often drain away vital morning energy. Just as you would want to warm up you motor and get the kinks out of your car before taking it on the road, so should you warm up the tight and kinky muscles of your neck in order to benefit from a fresh flow of oxygen-carrying energy. The Head Circler helps relax the neck and ease

tense, sore muscles. To practice, just stand (or sit) with hands on your hips. Breathe in—and slowly circle your head to the left and straight back. Breathe out—and circle your head to the right and back. Relax and continue the circle by dropping your chin onto your chest. Complete another circle to your left and pause with your chin on your chest. Breathe in and raise your head as if to look up. Breathe out and drop your chin back to your chest. To conclude: relax and pause and circle your head to the right. Repeat just four times. *Note:* you should feel a pleasant pull as you stretch those tensed-up neck and shoulder muscles.

RELAX YOUR WAY TO BETTER ENERGY. The preceding seven natural laws of self-energy help oxygenate your system, flush out wastes and invigorate your mind and body. You may want to perform them before a mirror for "company" and at the same time you can coach yourself. To benefit, you should follow these laws every morning. An occasional, hit-or-miss program will not give you the energy-producing benefits you seek. After you fit them into your schedule, they should require just ten golden minutes in the morning that add up to ten golden hours of better energy!

The Natural Laws of Refreshing Sleep With Hydrotherapy

Benefits of Water Healing. The ancients and moderns know the benefits of soothing water to provide healthful sleep. If you feel tired and tense, a comfortably warm bath can provide a natural tonic. It is known to be one of the oldest and best remedies for loosening muscle kinks. By dilating the blood vessels and soothing the circulation, a warm bath helps nourish the part of the body that seeks help. In most situations, it brings immediate relief and eases stress and tension.

The Wrong Way to Take a Bath. Frances T. wanted to give up her costly and dizzying tranquilizers. She heard, rightfully so, that a comfortably hot bath can be a natural sedative to quiet the nervous system. So she would heat up a tub of water, dunk herself, splash around and then get out. She was just as nervous as ever. Sleep was elusive. Frances T. gave up on the idea of hydrotherapy. Actually, she learned that there is a right way—and a wrong way— to take a bath!

Basic Law of a Refreshing Bath. To benefit from hydro-therapy, take a lukewarm bath before getting into bed where you perform your breathing exercises. You fill your bath tub "full" so that only your head is above water. The temperature should be mildly warm to the skin. Lie back. Soak yourself up to 20 or 30 minutes. Close your eyes. Rest your head against a rubber neck pillow. Let yourself go limp. See that bathroom lights do not shine in your eyes. Splash away the cares from your mind as you relax. Afterwards, pat yourself *gently* dry with a soft towel, climb into bed, breathe your way to a refreshing night's sleep.

THE SOOTHING ALKALINE BATH. The benefit of this warm bath is that it provides a nerve-soothing relaxation. Many problems of sleeplessness may be traced to overactive nerves. We know that the entire skin surface of the body is covered with nerve fibers. The soothing alkaline bath creates warmth in the network of nerves which, in turn, are connected to body organs. By soothing the nerves, the alkaline bath helps relax the connected body organs. This bath also promotes a healthful perspiration that casts off abrasive infectious matter such as urea and carbon dioxide. This washes the nerves and creates body organ relaxation.

How to Take an Alkaline Bath. Fill the tub three-quarters full of water at neutral temperature (90°-94° F.) and add one pound of ordinary baking soda. Stir vigorously to dissolve. Immerse yourself. If you wish, place a cold compress (cloth wrung out of cold water—60° F.) around the throat to avoid cerebral congestion. A rubber collar and cap which are more easily handled, may be used; fill with cold water or cracked ice and place on the neck and head at the start of the bath. Remain immersed up to half an hour. The soothing alkaline bath has been found to benefit those with nerves that tingle on the surface of the skin. It is also beneficial by applying a mild sedative action on the entire body surface.

THE AROMATIC BATH. This time-tested sleep-inducing bath is one in which pine needle oil, oil of eucalyptus or other aromatic oils (available at most pharmacies or cosmetic shops as well as health stores) are added to the bath water. The water temperature is from 93°-98° F. Fill the tub and immerse yourself up to 20 minutes. The aromatic bath is beneficial because of its refreshing fragrance and its soothing effect on nervous, high-strung people.

THE SALINE BATH. The tub is filled approximately three-quarters full of water, at a temperature of 90°-94° F. Dissolve one to two pounds of coarse salt into the water. Soak yourself in this tub for up to 15 minutes. Drink water in order to help increase a flow of perspiration. Afterwards, wash off with clear water. *Benefit of saline bath:* This particular folk remedy helps relax muscle fibers. It dilates the surface of the blood vessels, and lessens the viscosity of the blood which helps the blood pass from the arteries through the capillaries and into the veins with lessened effort required from the heart. This creates internal washing and harmony that promotes refreshing sleep—*without effort!*

THE WHEAT BRAN BATH FOR HEALING NERVES. Johanna E., faced with the pressures of holding down a job and managing a home at night, found the going too rough. If only she could enjoy a healthful night of sleep! But as soon as she crawled into bed, she felt a sensation of "little ants" climbing up and down her body. Her nerves had gotten the best of her and kept her tossing and turning until dawn. She was too tensed up to try the Basic Air Bath. She wanted "instant help" from the Seven Natural Laws of Morning Pep. She sought a compromise with Nature and lost out on lost sleep. But she did try a time-tested folk healer—the wheat bran bath. Here is what helped Johanna E. relax herself to sleep:

The Benefits of the Wheat Bran Bath: Through the addition of two pounds of wheat bran (or cornstarch or malt) to a tub of water with a warmth of 94°-96° F., a soothing reaction resulted that helped ease the "crawly" nerve irritation to the skin. Johanna soaked herself in this bath for 30 minutes. The wheat bran bath caused an increase in the number of leucocytes (white blood cells) in the skin. These leucocytes then rushed to help soothe the abrasive nerves. This relaxed Johanna. Furthermore, the wheat bran bath relaxed her muscles, soothed the voluntary and involuntary muscular systems. It relieved fatigue caused by tension-muscle exertion, driving the toxins of fatigue from the muscle area and helping to create natural relaxation. Just 30 minutes eased Johanna's tension and she could enjoy partial sleep. Yes, only partial because since she followed only one natural law she derived just that portion of benefit.

How Fomentations Help Relax Tight Muscle Spots

Andrew T. was troubled with local tension that afflicted the back of his neck, sometimes his shoulders, the small of his back or his spine. He was a systematic engineer and spent long hours over a drawing board. Realizing that his posture was slumped, he tried corrective exercises regularly to help ease congestion. But Andrew T. found that even after he used breathing exercises and followed other natural laws, he still felt a tight knot in his back that interfered with sleep. He was told to try a simple and effective sleep-inducer known as *fomentations.*

Relax Sore Spots with Fomentations. A fomentation is simply a hot local pack. It is applied to the tense, congested area where it helps relax and soothe the tight-as-a-knot feeling. Andrew T. used an ordinary large bath towel. He soaked it in hot water. To "seal in" the heat, he wrapped this with another towel that was dry. He then applied it directly to the back of his neck or the spinal region that was tight and gnarled. He let it remain up to 20 minutes. He felt a gradual lifting of knotted tensions. Slowly, with repeated fomentations, he was able to melt away the clogged trouble spots and now he could relax into a refreshing sleep.

Since muscular tension (a symptom of emotional upset) manifests itself in localized regions, the fomentation will be beneficial for reducing a feeling of inflammation, in the dispersal of congestion and to help regulate a soothing and healthful blood pressure.

The Natural Law of Tension Melting: Since the ten minutes *before* going to sleep are the most valuable, it is most beneficial to fit a soothing bath into the pre-sleep schedule. Begin about an hour before you retire. Put everything in order, then take your selected relaxing bath. During the final ten minutes, in bed, self-ventilate yourself with the breathing programs and create a soothing sleep environment that helps you go to sleep refreshed!

The Natural Sleep Law of the Healthy American Indians

A group of volunteer workers went among the American Indians to help them improve their living conditions. The non-Indian volunteers noted that there was virtually little problem with insomnia. True, the fresh air, the mountain tranquility, the absence of constant tension would promote soothing sleep. But the non-Indian volunteers lived in the same environment yet had civilized insomnia! It was after prolonged investigation that they learned the American Indians had a traditional law about sleeping which promoted natural sleep with little effort.

The American Indian Sleeping Law: The most favored sleeping position is the one on the right side because while you are in this position, the work of the heart, lungs and the stomach is relaxed since they are on top of the other inner organs in this position. The American Indians may have learned this health law from generations of medicine men or spiritual healers and they still follow it in our modern times. They enjoy refreshing sleep by sleeping on the right side. It is believed they are trained to use the right side from early childhood.

The volunteer workers tried the same method and some of them reported it helped give them a deep and satisfying sleep. But others concentrated too deeply on getting to sleep. They erred by working at going to sleep, which created more tension and resultant insomnia. The American Indian may well have the solution to insomnia with this traditional natural law of sleeping on the right side without any effort or emotional concentration.

BENEFITS OF A NAP BEFORE YOU GO TO SLEEP. A charged-up brain and nervous system has to be relaxed before it can let you sleep. To jump into bed, unprepared, is like roaring up your car's motor without advance warning. You let yourself in for a lot of trouble. If you can take a brief nap a few hours before established bedtime, you help relax your brain and nervous system. You therefore prepare yourself for refreshing sleep, just as you should prepare your car's motor with gentle persuasion for a long drive ahead.

Progressive Relaxation for Overall Contentment. If you can't relax immediately, then try it in progressive stages. Divert your thoughts from business and family worries. Instead, concentrate on small portions of your body, one at a time. For example, "Right little finger, relax! Right ring finger, relax! Right middle finger, relax!" Do this with each finger of each hand in regular progression. Then do it with each toe of each foot. Then go upward and relax all the joints and slowly relax your chest, your back, your individual muscles, your neck and your head, your nostrils, your eyelids. In progressive stages, you can relax and thus create a contentment for a refreshing nap. When you awaken from your nap, the melted tensions create a state of euphoria that is a natural sleep-inducer when you finally get into bed at your scheduled bedtime. Otherwise, if you plunge right into bed, you may fall asleep and then awaken and toss and turn all night long. So take your nap *before* you go to bed!

THE NATURAL LAW OF EYE RELAXATION. Researchers have found that much sleeplessness is traced to *staring* even when the eyelids are shut! Tension can cause this unhealthful condition. A natural law of eye relaxation is to use part of your Ten Golden Minutes *before* going to bed to relax yourself with simple water. Apply comfortably hot water to the closed eyes. Follow with an application of comfortably cold water. This helps flush out impurities and also dilates clogged arteries. The natural law is beneficial since it promotes circulation to sluggish channels that force the eye to stare wide open even though the lids are closed in craved-for sleep!

The Waerland Law of Healthful Sleep

The natural healer of Sweden, Are Waerland, affirmed that refreshing sleep is the great natural law. He felt it came first in the program of abundantly healthful living since sleep was the way the body recuperated and regenerated itself. Among some of his laws for healthful sleep are these natural methods:

1. Air should be comfortably cool in the sleeping environment. Breathing through the nose will warm the air that is taken in; yet cold air provokes deep breathing which, in turn, is conducive to sleep. It might be that the nose, on the passage of the cold air, by means of the nerves coaxes the lungs to take in more fresh oxygen. Are Waerland treated many insomniacs by prescribing that they sleep in a comfortably cold room.

2. The Waerland law adds that in addition to cold fresh air which is favorable for breathing during sleep, there are also the good smells of Nature. He suggested opening windows to permit the sleep-inducing fragrances of the trees, grass, garden plants, new fallen snow. Waerland, himself, preferred sleeping in the open air and rarely had insomnia. He went to sleep—and awakened—totally refreshed.

3. The Waerland law for starting off the day properly is to take a brisk walk after rising. He found that the motion of the muscles would invigorate the bloodstream and stimulate the body with oxygen, which is most essential for refreshment.

How Herbs Help Cause Natural Sleep

For those who would like to look to Nature's medicines from the meadows for a healthful herbal tonic, we dip into folklore and find this *Herbal Night Cap:*

Select *one* of these herbs: lady's slipper, valerian, scullcap or hops.

Use one teaspoonful of any *one* of the above herbs. Steep in a cup of boiling water for 20 minutes. Drink while comfortably hot. This Herbal Night Cap will reportedly soothe the stomach and nerves and promote a feeling of gentle euphoria and gradual sleep.

FRUIT JUICE NIGHT CAP. If you do not have herbs on hand, hot lemonade (sour) or hot grapefruit juice is reportedly a most beneficial night cap. Minerals in the juice help nullify frazzled nerves and promote a relaxation from tension and gradual lulling into sleep.

TWO TEN-MINUTE PROGRAMS TO PROMOTE HEALTHFUL SLEEP. A wise man once said, "He who would be healthy in the morning must prepare like the camel at bedtime to have his burdens lifted. For to the unburdened, the night will be filled by pleasant dreams, tender, refreshing, healing dreams, bright as stardust. For sleep is a gentle maid, beautiful as an angel, who brings her lovely wares for the one who rests without fear or anxiety, safe and secure."

The first ten-minute program helps promote refreshing sleep. The second ten-minute program of morning energizers helps you meet the new day with courage and confidence. Altogether—20 golden minutes. If you use them effectively, they will condition your life and make you a dynamic, energetic, confident, and amazingly healthfully happy person!

Highlights of Chapter 18:

1. Two ten-minute periods can influence your entire day. Make the most of them to help promote refreshing sleep and morning energy.

2. A simple deep breathing program helps promote refreshing sleep without drugs.

3. Start the day with the easy seven natural laws of morning pep that can be followed in just ten minutes. Ralph H., a highly successful businessman, keeps up with younger competition with this invigorator of mind and body.

4. The Basic Air Bath helps promote refreshing energy.

5. Simple baths can help promote muscle relaxation and a natural sleep. Try the alkaline, aromatic, saline, wheat bran bath.

6. Fomentations ease tight muscle spots and help promote tranquility.

7. The American Indians offer a secret sleeping technique that provides refreshing sleep—the natural way.

8. The Waerland Laws, healing herbs and fruit juice are all natural ways for sleep rejuvenation.

19

HOW TO USE HERBS AS NATURE'S POWERHOUSES OF HEALING

In the days before drugs were invented, healing was performed through natural medications. High on the list of natural healing laws were *herbs.* Ancient healers compiled from the meadows, massive directories of these herbs, these healing grasses, these *drugless medicines.* In due time, there were herbs prescribed for virtually all emotional and physical problems. Throughout the centuries, herbs have always been used for the restoration and boosting of health. Today, herbs are again enjoying a rebirth and are a blessing for those who seek natural and drugless healing.

THE NATURAL LAWS OF HEALING HERBS. Basically, herbs offer the following benefits: they relieve pain, cause natural digestive regularity, act as a natural stimulant, internal washing, restoration of metabolism and other vital body processes, counteract effects of putrefaction, promote healing, soothe and relieve inflammation, purify the blood, cleanse skin disorders, dissolve plaques, cause natural fever, soften and soothe inflamed parts, promote health of internal organs, act as a natural refrigerant or cooling agent, pep up circulation, stabilize nervous system, cause invigoration and strengthening. The *basic benefit* is in the natural healing power of herbs. We are fortunate in knowing that there are close to one thousand known herbs that help provide healing for virtually all known disorders. In the following list, some of the more prominent herbs are listed. To obtain herbs, inquire at your nearest herbal pharmacy. Look in the classified telephone directory for names and addresses of these pharmacies. •

How to Use Herbs

Granulated or finely cut herbs. Steep a heaping teaspoon of selected herbs in a cup of boiling water for 20 minutes. Strain. Take 1 cup an hour before each meal and 1 cup upon retiring. Take more or less as the case requires. If too strong, reduce the amount of herbs per cup. *Roots and barks.* Roots must be simmered 30 minutes or more in order to extract their natural medicinal value. Do not boil hard. *Flowers and leaves.* These should never be boiled. Instead, steep them in boiling water in a covered dish for 20 minutes, just as you would make tea. Boiling evaporates the aromatic properties. *Powdered herbs.* The powdered herbs may be mixed in hot or cold water. Use ½ teaspoon to ¼ glass of water. Follow by drinking 1 glass of water, either hot or cold. Herbs usually take effect quicker if taken in hot water. Powdered herbs may also be mixed with foods such as mashed potatoes or mashed vegetables of any kind, or sweet fruits, such as figs or dates, ground. *Herbal syrups.* To make, simply add the cut herbs (or if using granulated herbs, sift them so there will not be dust or sediment), boil to a syrupy consistency and strain through a double cheesecloth. Bottle for repeated use.

HOW TO MAKE HERB SALVES. Use fresh leaves, flowers, roots, barks or the dried granulated or powdered herbs. If you gather the herbs yourself, be sure to use them fresh and cut them up finely. Use 1 pound of herbs to 1½ pounds of any pure vegetable fat and 4 ounces beeswax. It is necessary to use a little more beeswax in a warmer climate as this ingredient keeps the salve firm. Mix the above together. Cover. Place in the oven, with the fire turned low, for three hours. Strain through a fine sieve or cloth. When cold, the herb salve will be firm and ready for use. It may be used, however, before it is cold.

HOW TO MAKE HERB POULTICES. Select herbs in a ground or granulated form. For ground or powdered herbs, mix with just enough water to make a thick paste. When using granulated herbs, mix with water, cornmeal or flaxseed meal to make a thick paste. If fresh green leaves are used, beat them up, steep and apply to the affected parts.

Adele S. was troubled with recurring blotches on her face and throat. She tried expensive medications which caused severe itching and inflammation. She might have given up, erroneously assuming that "old age spots" and "old age blemishes" were just part of getting old! But she learned that Nature has a law that helps promote self-healing and prolonged youth. She tried several all-herb poultices and was able to relieve the itching, soothe inflammation and bring down her unsightly skin eruptions and boils. She had used a slippery elm poultice, having obtained this granulated herb at a local herbal pharmacy. Other herbs could be beneficial as well. Now Adele S. looked and felt better. Her skin was young and fresh and herbal-healthy!

Herbal Health and Beauty Guide

FEVER. The powdered root of the American hellebore is useful as a tea and also soothing as a gargle for a sore throat.

MOUTH SORES. The seed of the common columbine is reportedly soothing to mouth, tongue and gum inflammations and disorders. It is also good as a gargle. Use as a tea for sipping daily, as well as for a mouth wash and gargle.

BOWEL REGULATION. A tea made of St.-John's-wort is said to be a natural astringent and also a diuretic.

HEALTH BOOSTER. A tea made of the powdered root of goldthread is said to improve the appetite, promote digestion and act as a general stimulant to the body. It also soothes irritation of the mouth and lips.

BLOOD BUILDING. The herb and root of the sweet cicely are said to correct conditions of anemia. The fresh root eaten freely has been said to soothe coughs and also stimulate digestion. It is regarded as a blood-building herb tonic for those with chilled hands and feet.

NERVOUS TREMORS. The seeds of the cedron made into a

tea are reportedly said to soothe spasms, dyspepsia and nervous disorders.

YOUTH RESTORATION. Legend has it that the leaves of the damiana plant, made into a tea, help promote a feeling of vitality and youth. It is reported to bestow a general and beneficial action upon the vital organs. It creates a feeling of youth, according to herbalists.

ARTHRITIS DISTRESS. The whole herb of the lucerne or alfalfa is regarded as soothing for problems of rheumatism-arthritis. One victim of gnarled joints and twisted limbs, Earl T., found that his distress was eased when he took 1 teaspoon of powdered lucerne and 1 teaspoon of powdered alfalfa with cider vinegar and honey in water. He took 3 cups of such tea daily. But while Earl T. could now bend his fingers to hold a pencil, he was still ailing because he disregarded the other natural laws of healing. Again we see that you derive as much benefit as you put into your program. Follow just one law (such as herbal healing) and you benefit with that one portion of the natural laws of abundantly healthful living.

ASTHMATIC DISORDER. The root of the butterbar is said to facilitate breathing. It reportedly helps conditions of respiratory disorder, helps promote better lung health and also "carries" a precious flow of oxygen throughout the entire breathing apparatus. A delicious tea that is as healing good as it tastes!

BEAUTY HERB. The entire herb of the frostwort or rockrose is soothing for creating a youthful skin. Pliny, the ancient herbalist-author, reported that when the ancients would anoint their bodies with a salve made of either of these two herbs, they would "seem fair and beautiful." These herbs may also be made into a tea to promote inner beauty!

CRAMPS. The entire herb of allheal or woundwort is said to soothe churning stomach. It may be made into a syrup or tea, or apply boiled leaves to the affected throbbing region for external poultice soothing.

YOUTHFUL JOINTS. The noted herbalist-researcher, Culpepper, writes, "A decoction of the leaves of Sage, Marjoram and Camomile Flowers and the places bathed therewith that have the sinews stiff with cold or cramp doth bring much ease and comfort." Another legendary herbalist, Gerard, urged the application of the leaves and flowers of the herb, mullein, to cramped wrists, ankles, knees and other body parts to make them youthful and flexible.

BLACK AND BLUE MARKS ON SKIN. In Culpeper's Herbal book we read, "The leaves or bark of the Bay Tree do dry and heal very much. The oil takes away the marks of the skin and flesh by bruises, falls, etc., and dissolves the congealed blood in them. It helps also the itch, scabs and weals in the skin."

BLADDER AND KIDNEY COMPLAINTS. The entire parsley herb used as tea is said to act directly on the kidney and other affected parts. Many London physicians prescribe parsley tea quite regularly. It is said to regulate bladder function.

BURNS. According to the ancient herbal-healer, John Parkinson, "the leaves of the Burdock herb, being bruised with the white of an egg and laid on any place burnt with fire doth take out the fire, giveth sudden ease and heals it up afterwards." It is also said to be internally soothing to conditions of digestive "burning" or hyperacidity. The root and seed, either or both, may be used to prepare a healing tea.

SCURVY. The entire brooklime is said to nourish the blood and remove impurities, It is also claimed that a tea of the brooklime herb has the ability to pulverize bladder stones and pass the gravel away.

BODY HEAT GENERATOR—COLDNESS OF EXTREMITIES. The bayberry bark, made into a tea, is said to be one of the most useful and beneficial herbs in botanic "medicure." The ingredients in this herb help create a natural blood and circulatory stimulant. An "always cold" librarian, Grace Y., had to wear a sweater even in warm weather. She caught colds throughout the year, even in the summertime! Grace Y. tried "blood builders" but the combination of drugs made her sick and drowsy and did not make her feel naturally warm. She tried drinking bayberry bark tea and in conjunction with other natural laws such as hydrotheraphy and corrective diet, was able to boost circulation and bring desired warmth to her extremities. She caught occasional colds but she feels that in time, as she continues natural corrective healing, she will be immune to winter distress. Bayberry has the ability to "turn on" the body's own radiator system.

BRONCHIAL DISORDERS. The seeds and leaves of the sunflower, when made into an herbal tea, are said to provide a soothing relaxation for problems of bronchitis, laryngitis and pulmonary distress.

BRUISES AND SWELLINGS. For *external use only*, the stem and flowers of the arnica are said to be soothing as a poultice. This herbal plant is one of the most widely used in homeopathy for such varied conditions as neuralgic pains, pains caused by overstrain of muscles, sinews and joints, spinal paralysis, intermittent fever, concussion, chilblains, bruises and swelling.

EYEWASH. Cineraria maritima, native to the West Indies, but available in other parts of the world (including the United States), is reported to be eye-soothing. The juice of the plant is to be used after it is properly sterilized. It may be used as an eyewash to relieve itching, inflammation and a feeling of tired eyesight. Many herbal pharmacies have the cineraria maritima in a juice form, ready for use. It is also known as dusty miller.

CATARRH. The natives of India use the fresh leaves of the benne plant by steeping in water and then drinking its mucilaginous juice freely. It is said to be soothing to conditions of catarrh, diarrhea, affections of the kidney and bladder. A missionary, Edward T., reports that he suffered from recurring skin disorders as well as chronic catarrh until his Hindu servant gave him a tea of the benne plant and this helped heal his throat and nose distress. His skin was treated to a poultice made of benne leaves and he related that his blemishes cleared up.

CHAPPED SKIN. The sanicle herb, made into a poultice or salve, is said to cause a natural astringent beneficial to the problem of rough, chapped skin. Country people use it to anoint their hands when bruised or chapped by the sun, wind or much water exposure.

CHEST, LUNG, STOMACH AND KIDNEY COMPLAINTS.

The balm of Gilead has been highly rated since time immemorial. The buds are used in making an ointment to soothe wounds, scalds, gout, hemorrhoids and even for the promotion of hair growth! When applied to the external affected region and massaged gently, the balm of Gilead provides a soothing and gently healing benefit.

CONSTIPATION. The stem of the blackroot, made into a powder and used as a tea, is said to be able to cause a natural bowel movement. It is regarded as a soothing and all-natural herbal laxative.

COLD SORES AND WINTER DISTRESS. The whole plant of the true and common dulse is said to be extremely soothing when applied as a poultice to a cold sore. For treatment of colds, made into a tea, it is second to none. It is claimed to contain more than 300 times more iodine than wheat, and 50 times more iron than most known foods. The Scots and Maritimers avoid wintry distress by eating the dried dulse as others would eat a stick of celery or lettuce leaves.

COMPLEXION BOOSTER. A not-too-well known herb, the goa (araroba or chrysarobin, originally from Brazil) has long been used by European healers to improve the complexion. The goa powder is mixed with vinegar, lemon juice or glycerine to form a paste; then it is used as an ointment for the skin. It heals blemishes and causes a bloom of youth, according to European herbalists.

LAXATIVE NEED. The pulp of the cassia pod, usually combined with the senna herb, taken in small quantities, is said to provide a natural laxative action.

HERBAL COUGH MEDICINES. The leaves of the coltsfoot, used with other herbs such as horehound, marshmallow, ground ivy, in a tea form, sweetened with honey, is a most soothing herbal cough remedy.

EXCESS BLOOD SUGAR. For conditions that resemble diabetes, herbal pharmacists have time-tested healing methods. The seeds of the jambul herb, when made into a tea, are said to reduce the amount of sugar present in urine. Also, the periwinkle herb, when made into a tea, is reported as being able to cause a natural assimilation of excess sugar in the blood stream.

DRY, HACKING COUGH. Here is a herbal medicine used with much success among London healers: "Take a large teaspoonful of linseed oil, 1 ounce of licorice root, and ¼ pound of best raisins. Put them into 2 quarts of water and simmer down to 1 quart. Then add 1 tablespoon of white wine vinegar, several tablespoons of natural organic honey. Drink 2 cups when going to bed. Take a little whenever the cough is troublesome."

DYSPEPSIA (Poor digestion). The brilliant herbalist, Culpeper, suggested that the herb and leaves of the centaury be made into a tea and sipped throughout the day. He said it boosted enzymatic flow and caused a natural digestion. It has a pungent taste and may be sweetened with a little honey.

CORNS AND WARTS. The fresh juice of the celandine herb has long been used for the easing of painful corns and warts. Apply to the affected region and let remain until dry.

HERBAL ELIXIR. The slippery elm is known to be one of the most beneficial of herbs. It offers a variety of uses. *Food:* Take 1 teaspoon of slippery elm powder, mix well with 1 teaspoon of raw sugar and add 1 pint of boiling water slowly, mixing as it is poured on. Use as a pep-up Herbal Elixir. *Poultice:* The coarse powder of slippery elm forms a soothing poultice for inflamed surfaces, wounds, burns, boils, skin diseases, chilblains, etc. It reportedly soothes the part, melts the inflammation, draws out impurities and speeds healing.

INFLAMMATION—FEVER DISORDERS. A variety of herbs have always been used to create a cooling of inflammation-fever problems. The fruit and pulp of the tamarind makes a soothing tea. The whole balm helps induce a mild perspiration and creates a pleasant and cooling tea. The stem of the berberis, as a tea, is used in India as a bitter tonic in intermittent fevers.

FRECKLES, SPOTS AND PIMPLES ON THE FACE. The herbalist, Gerard, wrote, "The juice of Silverweed takes away freckles, spots, pimples on the face, and sunburning. The best of all is to steep Silverweed in strong white wine vinegar, the face being often bathed or washed therewith."

UPSET NERVES. The flower of the camomile, made into tea, is soothing to the nervous system. It is best known as a poultice, when combined with crushed poppy heads, applied externally to aching parts.

INSOMNIA. When the gelsemium root is used in small doses for a tea, it is reportedly soothing to the system, It is said to help promote a natural desire for sleep.

INTESTINAL LUBRICANT. The seeds of the psyllium offer a mucilaginous, bulking benefit. When moistened, the psyllium seeds swell into a gelatinous mass, which stimulates and lubricates the intestinal tract. To prepare, place psyllium seeds in boiled water, stir until the mixture thickens, then drink. Add a little lemon juice to make more palatable.

NOCTURNAL INCONTINENCE. This problem is one faced by many men with prostatic disorders and women in the more mature years; they have to wake up frequently for bathroom trips. The herbalists suggested the root of the kavakava herb as a mild tea. It reportedly was able to strengthen the bladder.

PILES OR HEMORRHOIDS. A physician writes that the entire herb, pilewort, macerated in boiling lard and then used as an ointment for piles, applied locally twice daily, helps ease itching and promote relief.

HAIR RESTORER. The ancients suggested the use of rosemary, made into a tonic, combined with borax, and applied to the scalp. It was said to be able to stop falling hair, promote new growth. It is also good as a hair wash.

WRINKLES AND PREMATURE AGING. The seeds or groats of oat groats are to be made into a tonic and sipped throughout the day. Make a few small bags from cheese cloth. Fill with oatmeal. Use as a soap-substitute. Do not rinse the skin for five minutes after this herbal face wash. Let dry. Now rinse with cool water containing a few drops of tincture of benzoin. This herbal remedy will reportedly tighten up the skin and firm out furrows and wrinkles.

HERBS FORM THE FOUNDATION FOR ABUNDANTLY HEALTHFUL LIVING. As reported drugless medicines and healers from the woods and forests, herbs form the basic foundation for abundantly healthful living. They have been used since the dawn of the world, and today they are being used again in the quest for natural healing and health restoration.

Summation of This Chapter

1. Herbs have been used since the earliest records of history. They served as medicines and healers for virtually all disorders of the mind and body. They are known as drugless medicines!

2. Obtain desired herbs and grasses from any herbal pharmacy and perpare them at home for the desired health correction.

3. Seek Nature's grasses for your drugless medicines, as did the ancients who enjoyed abundantly healthful living.

20

NATURE'S HINTS FOR COPING WITH COMMON AND UNCOMMON HEALTH SITUATIONS

The basic Natural Law is to create an alliance with Nature, to stimulate and promote the body's built-in sources of self-healing. The key to healthful-plus living is in corrective diet, all-natural programs and drugless healing. Many of these health laws were known to the Persian and Greek sages. The wise healers of the Medieval Ages and the herbalists-nutritionists of the past century, all knew of the natural laws of abundantly healthful living. Today, we draw upon their knowledge and discoveries as well as folk remedies and time-tested healers for this chapter of home health hints. The benefit here is that most of these home health hints are absolutely cost-free! Many others use ordinary foods available in most market outlets. Nearly all are drug-free. These home health hints represent hundreds of centuries of secrets of drugless healers and are every bit as good today as they were in the days of all-natural healing.

EXTRA-HEALTH THROUGH NATURAL LAWS. To benefit from extra health, to tap the hidden wellsprings of youth and vitality within the body, to regenerate and restore precious good feeling, the natural laws are available for your use. The decision is yours. If a short and ailing life is preferred, you are at liberty to do as you like; but please remember, that if you "sow wind, you reap the whirlwind." If you violate Nature's laws, you pay for it in lost health, lost years of precious life. You now stand on the crossroads of life. Follow the Natural Laws for a long, healthy, youthful life. Here is your road map to a long, productive and energetic lifespan.

BREATHE RIGHT AND LIVE LONGER. Proper breathing rids the lungs of accumulated impurities. Better aeration of the lungs relieves bronchitis, respiratory and related ailments. One time-tested folk hint calls for breathing in to the count of 4, and out to the count of 12, then increasing the count until you are able to breathe in to 7 and out to 21. Each sequence should be repeated three times. The benefit is to flush out toxic wastes, to cast off stagnant plaques, to cause reawakening of energy sources. The benefit of this simple exercise is to reduce fatigue, woo sleep, create better feeling. Fill your lungs with life-giving oxygen and live longer.

HOW BREATHING CAN BOOST ENERGY. When you have something heavy to lift, take a deep breath and note how much lighter the object becomes. As you go up a staircase, breathe *in* on two steps, breathe *out* on two steps. You'll be less winded at the top. Pant deliberately like a dog for a few minutes and you'll get your wind back in a jiffy. If you're cold, do the same thing and see how fast you warm up. In our cars, we don't tolerate choked gas lines, faulty carburetors or other such things that lead to poor engine performance. Yet we accept (unnecessarily) poor body performance caused by an inadequacy in the oxygen supply that is essential to the health and well-being of our trillions of cells. Corrective breathing can benefit with better health and better living.

APRICOT TONIC FOR BLOOD ENRICHMENT. Sun-dried apricots soaked in pineapple juice overnight help make more blood-building iron and copper of the apricot available. Your bloodstream needs iron and copper for life-giving oxygenation. This simple Apricot Tonic is an excellent morning stimulator and blood enrichment.

HOW PROPER SLEEPING POSTURE IMPROVES CIRCULATION. You will benefit from better sleep if you use a firm hard mattress, or place a board under a soft one. When you have pains in the neck, try sleeping *without* a pillow. When sleeping, keep the arms relaxed below the shoulder line. Your head may be pressing on the arms which can cause shoulder-arm pain. Don't cross the knees. Don't put one ankle over the other; these bad sleeping postures break the natural circulation of the blood. Get many hours of sound sleep before midnight to produce daisy freshness in the morning, and twice your vitality.

HOW PRUNES CAN STIMULATE MENTAL ENERGY. A dish of stewed prunes with plenty of fruit juice and 3 to 5 tablespoons of raw wheat germ topped with honey will help alert the brain. This combination of natural fruit sugar and organic minerals helps speed oxygen-energy to the millions of brain cells and stimulates mental energy. Try this Prune Dish for lunch to help relieve the afternoon brain fatigue slump.

WALK YOUR WAY TO LIMBER JOINTS. Walking is beneficial for "oiling" the joints. Walking brings the body muscles into play, stimulates the circulation and provides body tissues with vital energy. Walking regulates the glands, normalizes a high pulse and is soothing for heart health. The joints have little chance to become "rusty" when they are exercised through regular walking.

BATH BRUSH FOR GLOWING SKIN. The hardy Indians who knew nothing of soap, would have glowing healthy skin by washing in cool and even cold water. One Indian secret was to use a stiff brush (they made them from twigs and branches, but today these body brushes are available in health stores and supermarkets) that was scrubbed over the body. If you can acclimate yourself to comfortably cold water and then use a bath brush to dry yourself, it will help give a glow to your skin and a tingle to your energy.

BOOST DIGESTION WITH ENZYMES. Enzymes are found in all living substances and help bring about activated digestion. One prime source of enzymes is in raw fruits and vegetables and their prepared juices. To benefit from enzymes, here are time-tested tips:

1. Serve all fruits raw, whenever possible.
2. Eat most vegetables raw.
3. Serve raw foods first to stimulate digestive powers.

4. Since sprouting increases the enzymatic content of seeds and grains, try to serve sprouts daily.

HOW TO MAKE SPROUTS. Use either rye, wheat, any seeds, grains or nuts. Mung beans, when sprouted, contain an enzyme known as *auxim* that reportedly causes tissue and cellular rejuvenation. They are fed to burned out race horses to bring them back to record breaking running power. *How to sprout.* Use clean, bright new crop seeds. Soak overnight in a wide-mouthed mason jar. In the morning, drain, saving liquid for soups or broths or vegetable juices. Place the soaked seeds in the jar and cover the top with screen wire, cut to fit. Screw lid on tightly. Water under tap two or three times daily; turn on side in bowl or pan to drain or set completely upside down on two small boards to drain well. Grains will be best when the root is as long as the grain. Alfalfa and soy or other beans can be grown until the sprout is two or three inches long. You may use sprouts in salads, added to omelets, with fruit dishes, or just as is.

HOW TO CLEANSE THE LIVER FOR SELF–REBUILDING. The liver is the most important body organ concerned with protein metabolism. A healthy liver helps manufacture amino acids, detoxify poisonous substances, manage excess hormone secretions. To cleanse the liver, a natural food is raw beets. Another natural food for the liver includes beet greens. Raw organic cucumbers contain minerals and an enzyme that helps cleanse the liver. Here is a home health hint: *Liver Massage Exercise:* Lie on floor or on slant board, head down. Draw knees up to chest, hug with arms. Return feet out straight and hands over head. Repeat several times a day.

BURNS AND SCALDS. If you burn yourself with boiling water, ordinary icing sugar is said to be soothing and healing. If the burn is caused by hot oil or fat, cover it with flour to help ease the sting and promote natural healing.

SCRATCHES AND WOUNDS. A folk healer is to rinse the scratch or wound, then cover with a paste made of soaked wheat bran and milk. This helps promote self-healing. After two days, use pulped cabbage leaves as a poultice to help bring about total healing without any scars.

INFLAMED EYES. A well-known Swiss resort had complaints from tourists who suffered from eye inflammation caused by continuous exposure to the reflection of the sun on water or snow. They used a traditional drugless healer. They beat the white of an egg, spread it onto a cloth and bandaged it as a poultice over the eyes of the afflicted. It reportedly heals the inflammation overnight and also eases conditions of sun–blindness which may occur in the high mountains where there are large expanses of snow and ice.

NASAL CATARRH. It is reported that any seasonal berries eaten raw and uncooked will help relieve stubborn conditions of nasal catarrh.

VARICOSE VEINS. Also known as phlebitis, this condition was treated by folk healing by using an alcohol compress. When the inflammation was eased, a poultice of pulped cabbage leaves gave a soothing, relaxed feeling. In many reported situations, this folk healer program together with walking exercises was able to reduce varicose veins.

NATURAL HEART HEALTH TONIC. The naturopathic way of healing is for the heart-conscious person to chew dried currants and raisins slowly, throughout the day. It is believed that the minerals and vitamins and natural enzymes in these fruits are nutritious to the heart muscles. Naturopaths also maintain that relief from continuous heart pains can be obtained from the woody, interior dividing walls of *walnuts*. Boil these for a few minutes; cover the pan and let it stand for about ten minutes. This infusion is said to soothe the heart when sipped as a tea.

HEARTBURN. A much harried saleswoman, Louise D., finds that she suffers from excess acidity. The hyperacidity of her stomach is so bad that the acid rises into the mouth. She tried medications but bicarbonate of soda preparations dissolve the precious B-complex supply in the system and interfere with calcium metabolism. Louise D. then tried a simple home remedy that provided soothing relief. She grated raw potato, squeezed out the juice, diluted it with freshly poured water, and drank one cup first thing in the morning, another cup before lunch, and a last cup before retiring at night. The rich mineral supply and the high *natural* alkaline of the potato helped dilute and wash off the excess stomach acid. Now she felt light, sweet and refreshed. Nature promoted natural healing.

HEADACHE DISTRESS. Many a headache inflammation can be relieved by applying an onion or horseradish poultice to the neck, calves and the soles of the feet. The benefit here is to draw away the pounding blood from the head.

SKIN ITCHING. This is often referred to as *pruritis.* A home remedy is to rub the itching part with slices of raw potato. Or you can grate the potato finely and apply the pulp as a poultice. It is healthful to eliminate sharp condiments, salt and unnatural spices. Emphasize fresh fruit and vegetable juices. This helps wash out acid-forming substances that itch as they get through the skin.

PAINFUL SWELLING. Lena T. hurt her hand while lifting heavy kitchen pots. One finger swelled up. She feared having to put the entire hand in a cast. She hurried to a neighbor for help. The neighbor had her soak the finger in warm water (98-100° F.) three times a day, for an hour each time. If the water became cool, fresh hot water was poured to maintain the soothing penetrating heat of the water. Lena T. experienced relief. Soon the swelling subsided enough for her to eliminate this natural and drugless treatment. She had relied upon Nature and was rewarded with a natural healing of her swollen finger.

CLEANING THE KIDNEYS. The kidneys filter approximately 4,000 quarts of blood daily. It is important to have *clean* kidneys that are able to eliminate wastes such as urea and also to help maintain the acid-alkaline balance. Plenty of liquids should be taken. A good kidney-wash home remedy is the juice of one lemon in a cup of hot water, twice daily. Naturopaths suggest taking this throughout the winter. This helps promote a kidney-wash.

YOUTH-SKIN PROGRAM. It is reported that the Grecian beauties of ancient days had this program: after a soaking bath, they would rub the body from head to toe with a mixture of olive oil and castor oil in equal parts. They would again soak in a bath for 15 minutes to allow the oil to penetrate and then take a cleansing shower to wash off the oil and close the skin pores. The ageless youth-skin of the Grecian beauties attests to the wisdom of folk healing.

THE POWER OF RAW ALMONDS. Basic health is dependent upon enzymes from the pancreas. These enzymes build and nourish body cells and tissues. Raw almonds are a powerful source of pancreatic enzymes which will also serve as the body's cleansers inasmuch as they devour wastes and facilitate in their elimination. Whole raw almonds should be chewed slowly. For those who have difficulty in chewing, substitute pure raw almond butter, available in most health food stores.

The Natural Health Building Law of Green Food

Life energy comes from the sun. *Green plants* know the secret of how to capture this solar energy and pass it on to you. When you touch your body and feel warmth, that warmth came to you from the sun by green plants. Enzymes are juices of green plants that may be considered "plant blood." The Natural Law of Abundantly Healthful Living calls for the eating of green leaves. The benefits include:

1. Green raw leaves are rich in life-giving enzymes.

2. Green raw leaves carry an abundance of vitamins and minerals.

3. Green raw leaves are rich in valuable amino acids which complete the patterns of many "incomplete" proteins such as nuts, seeds, grains or beans which have had their amino acid pattern disturbed by heat.

4. Greens are alkaline in reaction to the body, thus favoring a healthful balance for good health.

5. Greens contain from 75 percent to 90 percent of pure Nature water.

6. Greens also contain bulk or fiber which becomes highly magnetized in its passage through the intestines, drawing from the body the discarded tissues and cell wastes, acting both as a broom and a vacuum cleaner. (When cooked, the action is like that of a mop, usually a slimy one; hence, the value of *raw* greens.)

The enzymes in green leaves help stimulate the bone marrow to produce hemoglobin; they enable the body to digest and utilize food, thus increasing resistance to sickness and aging. The enzymes in green leaves improve bowel action, normalize the heart, encourage tissue growth. The emphasis is on *raw green leafy vegetables.* You may enjoy them as a salad or as a "Green Drink," when put through a juicer or blender. If you must cook, then tenderize at the lowest possible temperature for the lowest possible time. But the Natural Law is for eating lots and lots of *raw* green leafy vegetables.

HOW TO PUT PROTEIN TO SUPER-USE IN YOUR BODY. The benefit of protein is to build the bloodstream, to perform the building of tissues and cells, to nourish, regenerate and replenish almost all that you can see and all that you cannot see. To put power into protein assimilation, a natural law calls for the use of *lysine*, a special enzyme that works with certain alkaline minerals including magnesium and potassium. *Lysine* is a spark plug that aids in the development of amino acids and also exerts a "dynamic" action to create protein-plus utilization in the body.

Where to get lysine: This enzyme is found in raw fresh vegetable juices, unroasted seeds, grains, nuts, soaked or sprouted and eaten raw or lightly cooked. For a powerhouse lysine source, mix equal potions of Brewer's yeast and wheat germ. Freeze in a vacuum sealed can and always keep under refrigeration. When you mix this Enzyme Tonic with some soya milk and add a sliced banana, you feed yourself a dynamic all-natural source of lysine that puts power into protein.

Rebuild Your Body with the Natural Laws of Life

The Natural Laws of Abundantly Healthful Living have been created to help you rebuild your body and your mind, the Nature way. As a child of Nature, you will benefit from her wise ways and reap the rewards of youthful health. When the Natural Laws are followed, you will benefit by getting younger and younger in accordance with successful assimilation.

There is an old saying, "Use it—or lose it!" This applies to your built-in and hidden wellsprings of natural health. Use these wellsprings of your own Fountain of Youth and enjoy abundantly healthful living. If you deny using them you may run the risk of losing this precious power of self-recuperation. The quest for health calls for reality through Nature's Laws. Once you have reaped the rewards you may well wonder why you waited so long. This book is your road map, your all-natural path to lasting good health and energetic youthfulness.

INDEX

A

Abdomen, water healing for, 168-169

Acid-alkaline balance, natural, restored by fever, 177
    ratio balanced by proper food combinations, 49

Acid fermentation, 57

Acid flow in stomach, regulation of by plant protein, 86-87

Acid mantle for skin, 39-40

Acid-starch combinations, 51

Adrenal glands, 127-128

Aerotherapy, 192

Age spots, use of cucumber juice for, 44-45

Aging digestion aided by papaya, 110

Air bath, natural law of, 192
    for morning pep, 214-215
    for proper ventilation, 137-138

"Air-washing" lungs by exercise, 142-143

Alkaline bath, 218

Alkaline Cocktail of Dr. Waerland, 95

Allergic, banana excellent food for, 104
    papaya excellent fruit for, 109-110

Allergies, self-defense against created by natural fever, 179-183

Allergies, using nature's laws to build immunities against, 134-143
    "air-washing" lungs by exercise, 142-143
    artificial carbohydrate foods, elimination of, 135
    condiments, sharp, avoiding, 139
    diet, basic, 135-136
    dry heat and chilling, 136-138
    inhalant, natural, 141
    laws, four natural, to "wash out," 138-139
    salt-free program, 141-142
    sinus distress relieved by corrective foods, 140-141
    Swiss all-natural healer, 139-140
    warm hands and feet, 139

"Alligator elbows," formula to prevent or correct, 40

Alligator pear as "miracle" health-building food, 100-103

Almonds, raw, power of, 241

"Almost-human" factor of papaya, 110

Aluminum utensils, relationship of to heart health, 162

American Journal of Orthodontics and Oral Surgery, 69

Amino acids in soybeans, benefits of, 111-112

Appetite, improvement of through raw foods, 31

Appetite control, avocado helpful in, 101
    banana excellent food for, 104-105

Apple as nature's magic miracle, 59-63

Apricot tonic for blood enrichment, 236

Aromatic bath, 218-219

Arterial health through proper feeding of thyroid, 148

Arteriosclerosis, avocado helpful in eliminating, 102

Artery function, how to help, 153-164
    Coronary-Youth Club, 157-159
    fat, 160-161
    folk laws, 162-163
    grains, whole, 159-160
    herbs, 162
    Lo-Carbo Heart-Youth Food Diet, 153-157
        program for health, 154-157
    rules for healthy heart, 161-162
    Vitamin E as supplier of air to heart, 160

Arthritic distress, paraffin bath for, 171-172

Avoeado as "miracle" health-building food, 100-103

B

Baby oil, benefits of for yourthful skin, 43

Back and shoulder breathing exercise, 210

Backache, bathing away, 172-173